In Clinical Practice

Taking a practical approach to clinical medicine, this series of smaller reference books is designed for the trainee physician, primary care physician, nurse practitioner and other general medical professionals to understand each topic covered. The coverage is comprehensive but concise and is designed to act as a primary reference tool for subjects across the field of medicine.

Neuseli Lamari · Peter Beighton

Hypermobility in Medical Practice

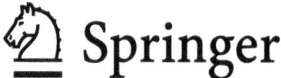 Springer

Neuseli Lamari
Faculty of Medicine of São José do
Rio Preto
São José do Rio Preto, Brazil

Peter Beighton
Faculty of Health Sciences
University of Cape Town
Cape Town, Western Cape
South Africa

ISSN 2199-6652 ISSN 2199-6660 (electronic)
In Clinical Practice
ISBN 978-3-031-34913-3 ISBN 978-3-031-34914-0 (eBook)
https://doi.org/10.1007/978-3-031-34914-0

This Springer imprint is published by the registered company Springer Nature
Switzerland AG
The registered company address is: Gewerbestrasse 11, 6330 Cham, Switzerland

In Memoriam of Professor Peter Beighton
In 2018, I had the honour and great fulfilment of personally meeting Prof. Beighton, who welcomed me to his home in Cape Town—South Africa. He introduced me to his library and presented me with relics of his productions, with the opportunity to appreciate all of his print productions. In these five uninterrupted years, with all his wisdom and knowledge, always added to ethical values, he helped me in each chapter of this book and even wrote exclusive chapters. Now we were already celebrating the completion of the book and scheduling our vernissage. Suddenly, he was gone, happy and fulfilled, leaving his last message: "our names will be linked to hyper-mobility for posterity". Of all the memories, the greatest was having known the essence of his concern for people affected by hypermobility. May these memories not only be mine, but may they also belong to all those who, directly or indirectly, were benefited by the contributions of the dear and immortal Prof. Beighton, who, for 59 years of his 89 years of life, devoted himself to people with hypermobility.

Neuseli Lamari

To my children,
Mateus and Mariana
and
To my great inspirer and best mentor,
Dr. Peter Beighton.

—Neuseli Lamari

To my children,
Charles, Robert and Victoria
and
To my grandchildren,
Edward, Olivia, Archie, Angus, Harry, Bella and Jamie.

—Peter Beighton

Preface: Elucidating the Ehlers-Danlos Syndrome

In 1966, I was a medical registrar training in internal medicine at St. Thomas's Hospital in London. I had passed the relevant higher examinations, and the next step on the academic ladder was a doctoral thesis. The great problem, however, was finding a suitable topic. The answer lay in the third edition of McKusick's magisterial monograph *Heritable Disorders of Connective Tissue* in which he provided dramatic illustrations of the articular and dermal manifestations of the Ehlers-Danlos Syndrome (EDS) and commented that only about 300 cases could be recognised in the world literature.

I had the good fortune to make a chance diagnosis of the EDS in a patient at St. Thomas's and presented case details at the weekly Grand Round. Three affected brothers were promptly referred to me by a kindly Consultant. I then realised if I could document the condition in a large series of affected persons in the UK, this would permit investigation of possible heterogeneity, the range of clinical manifestations and perhaps provide insight into the basic defect.

During my evenings on duty, I wrote to every orthopaedic surgeon and dermatologist in the south of England requesting access to any persons with the EDS in their care. When positive responses arrived I arranged to see the affected persons at St. Thomas's or if they lived away from London, I offered to visit them in their homes during my weekends off-duty. Now comes the nub of my story: In order to examine the patients I would need an assistant who could travel with me, act as a chaperone when necessary, record clinical and genealogical details and obtain biological specimens. Accordingly, I recruited a young nursing sister named Greta Janet Winch, and off we went.

At that time, when the world was real, and we were young, nothing could have exceeded the pleasure and joy of driving through the verdant English countryside in an open-topped sports car with this beautiful lady. Although we were happy because we were together and in love, at another level we were both very conscious of the duties and obligations inherent in our medical careers. We enjoyed excitement and laughter during our travels but there was also a deeper professional satisfaction in our contributions to medicine and humanity.

By the end of the year, I had seen and documented 100 persons with the EDS and analysis of the accumulated data began. The case details had been noted on standardised proformata, and for the sake of objectivity, the extent of the joint mobility was given a numerical notation. This was initially based upon orthopaedic investigations of dislocations and abnormal joint laxity (Carter and Wilkinson 1964) and was suggested by my close friend, Frank Horan FRCS. In essence, the movements of the fifth finger, wrist, elbow, knee and spine were assessed and a point was given for each site at which the range of joint mobility was excessive. This five-point score was subsequently used in other studies and depicted in the literature (Beighton and Horan 1969).

In 1968, I commenced a year as a research fellow at the Johns Hopkins Hospital, Baltimore, USA with Prof. V. McKusick. The exposure to his concepts and a large number of persons with genetic disorders who were encountered in his clinic were pivotal to my future career. While in Baltimore I mutated my Doctoral Thesis into a book on the EDS. Interest in hypermobility continued and the issue of familial joint laxity was addressed (Beighton and Horan 1970). Greta came with me to the USA and was a nurse at the "Big John". We had the opportunity to travel widely together in the USA with the result that our personal bonds became even closer.

We returned to the UK in 1969 and I departed to the Sahara Desert for a four-month research project with a British Para-Military Scientific and Exploration Expedition (Beighton 1971). I flew back from Algiers to Paris, where Greta and I had a brief romantic assignation. We then returned to England together and were married at last. On the following day, we sailed for South Africa in order to undertake an epidemiological investigation of bone joint disorders, including hypermobility in a rural Tswana community.

In South Africa, we joined the Department of Orthopaedic Surgery, University of Witwatersrand, Johannesburg. Greta was formally employed as my research associate, and we duly organised and completed the proposed investigation. The findings were analysed, documented and published. One of the articles concerned the assessment of joint mobility in several hundred persons in the community which we had studied. In the past, we had used a five-point score to quantitate the range of joint movements. During this new investigation in South

Africa, we used a nine-point score to document hypermobility as it had been realised that bilateral assessment of limb joints would be far more accurate than the unilateral approach that we had previously used (Beighton et al. 1973). With the nine-point score, it was possible to demonstrate a distinct age relationship with articular movements and there was also a lesser correlation with gender. This method for rapid assessment of an individual's joint movements subsequently came into general use under the eponymous designation "Beighton Score". But—the suggestion to use the nine-point score was made by my wife, Greta, and not by me. So eponymous immortality is rightly hers and not mine.

My beloved Greta with whom I worked and researched for more than fifty years died at the end of May 2017.

Cape Town, South Africa   Prof. Peter Beighton

References

Beighton P. Fluid balance in the Sahara. Nature. 1971;233(5317):275–277.

Beighton P, Horan F. Orthopaedic aspects of the Ehlers-Danlos syndrome. J Bone Jt Surg. 1969;51-B(3):444–453.

Beighton P, Horan F. Dominant inheritance in familial generalised articular hypermobility. J Bone Jt Surg. 1970;52-B(1):145–47.

Beighton P, Solomon L, Soskolne CL. Articular mobility in an African population. Ann Rheum Dis. 1973;32(5):413–418.

Carter CO, Wilkinson J. Persistent joint laxity and congenital dislocation of the hip. J Bone Jt Surg. 1964;46-B:40.

Acknowledgements

My gratitude to my son Mateus for the valuable content made available from his master's thesis and his doctoral thesis and in particular, my undying gratitude to Dr. Peter Beighton for years of intensive dedication to compiling this book.

—Neuseli Lamari

I offer my sincere gratitude to Deanah Lloyd for her expertise and generosity of spirit during the compilation of this book.

—Peter Beighton

We are also very grateful to Samantha Bayley for her diligent and competent secretarial assistance in the finalisation of the manuscript.

—Neuseli Lamari and Peter Beighton

Contents

Abbreviations

ACR-ARHP	American College of Rheumatology—Empowering Rheumatology Professionals
CBE	Commander of the Order of the British Empire
EDS	Elhers-Danlos Syndrome
EDS-HT	EDS Hypermobility Type
FAMERP	Faculty of Medicine of São José do Rio Preto
G-HSD	Generalised Hypermobility Spectrum Disorders
GJH	Generalised Joint Hypermobility
hEDS	Hypermobile Ehlers-Danlos Syndrome
H-HSD	Historical Hypermobility Spectrum Disorders
HMSA	Hypermobility Syndrome Association
HSDs	Hypermobility Spectrum Disorders
ILAR	International League of Associations of Rheumatology
JH	Joint Hypermobility
JHS	Joint Hypermobility Syndrome
L-HSD	Localised Hypermobility Spectrum Disorders
LJH	Localised Joint Hypermobilty

LPA	Little People of America
NL	Neuseli Lamari
P-HSD	Peripheral Hypermobility Spectrum Disorders
PJH	Peripheral Joint Hypermobility
SED BRASIL	Brazilian Association of Ehlers-Danlos Syndrome and Hypermobility
SP	São Paulo

About the Authors

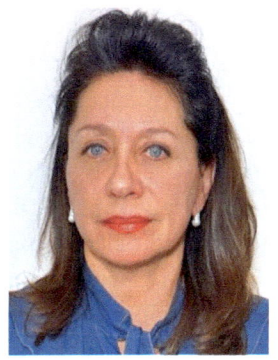

Prof. Neuseli Lamari (Physiotherapist) M.Sc., Ph.D. is a Research Scientist, Associate Professor in Health Sciences, and a Professional Physiotherapist with main focus on Joint Hypermobility and Ehlers-Danlos Syndromes. Currently, Neuseli Lamari is an Associate Professor and Senior Lecturer (Livre-Docente) in Health Sciences by the Faculty of Medicine of São José do Rio Preto (FAMERP), Brazil (2009).

Dr. Lamari has a Ph.D. in Health Sciences (2000) and a Master's degree (1994), both by FAMERP. Neuseli also has an undergraduate degree in Physiotherapy from the Methodist University of Piracicaba (UNIMEP), Brazil (1981). She is the founder of the Physiotherapy Service at the Hospital de Base of São José do Rio Preto (1984). It is a multidisciplinary teaching practice for undergraduate and graduate health students. The Physiotherapy Service is currently comprised of 275 physical therapists. In 1991, she implemented the Professional Enhancement Course in Physiotherapy as an in-service training at the Medical School Foundation of São José do Rio Preto (FUNFARME). Later in 2000, she implemented the Advanced Enhancement Training Course in Physiotherapy at FUNFARME.

In 1987, Dr. Neuseli implemented the Physiotherapy Service in Primary and Specialised Care with the Municipal Health Network of São José do Rio Preto. By 2022, this service involved 44 physical therapists and 135 professionals in various areas of physical, sensory and cognitive health promotion and rehabilitation.

Between 1989 and 1991, Neuseli conducted an important study with the Municipal Department of Education of São José do Rio Preto, which boosted her career. In this study, she analyzed 1120 children from 26 preschool units, as well as their families, comprising more than 5000 individuals. Dr. Lamari investigated Joint Hypermobility characteristics using the Beighton method. Her study was published in an *International Scientific Journal*.

Neuseli Lamari founded the first Multiprofessional Residency Program in Physical Rehabilitation in Brazil along with the Multiprofessional Residency Committee (COREMU—FAMERP), which is under her coordination since 2013. She was also responsible for the Joint Mobility discipline in the Stricto Sensu Graduate

Program of FAMERP. She has extensive experience in the Physiotherapy field with emphasis on Joint Hypermobility and Ehlers-Danlos Syndromes, as she has worked in this field for almost the entirety of her 40 years of professional practice.

In 2015, Dr. Lamari was awarded the July 19th Medal by the São José do Rio Preto City Council/Diploma of Gratitude in recognition for relevant services provided to the city, notably in physical and functional health recovery. She was also nominated as the first Rehabilitation Manager of the Municipal Health Department of São José do Rio Preto and had integral participation in the management of the Rehabilitation Network implementation in this municipality. Dr. Neuseli also implemented the first Brazilian "Emergency Unit in Physiotherapy" in 2014. As the recognised Brazilian expert in Hypermobility and Ehlers-Danlos Syndromes, she has given numerous interviews to the spoken and written media, including the highest-rated national networks.

Neuseli Lamari is the author and co-author of 40 full articles published in professional periodicals, she also published a book and 38 articles in newspapers and magazines. Besides, her career also includes 16 research works published in annals of scientific events and other journals and 43 research work presentations in conferences, lectures, congresses, and other scientific meetings. She has also contributed to 135 technical-scientific reviews; 79 scientific events, organisation of 21 scientific events and involvement in three examination committees and in 33 undergraduate and postgraduate conclusion work boards.

She has been a scientific advisor and has concluded 49 research projects of scientific initiation, undergraduate students, specialisations, and master's and doctoral degrees. Up to 2022, she has directly and indirectly contributed to approximately 50,000 hypermobile patients. Her indirect contributions include lectures for parents and teachers in elementary schools, universities, classes in undergraduate and graduate courses, conferences, seminars, congresses, lives, articles in newspapers and television news, comprising approximately 600 actions for knowledge dissemination concerning Hypermobility and the Ehlers-Danlos Syndromes.

In 2022, Neuseli was acknowledged by the "Rare Lives Institute" as one of the three health professionals in the category of "Rare Woman in Science/Rare Researcher" who most represent and work for rare diseases in Brazil. At the time of publication of this book, she was an Associate Professor and Senior Lecturer (Livre-Docente) at the Medical School of FAMERP, in the Department of Neurological Sciences, Psychiatry and Medical Psychology. She was also the general coordinator of the Multiprofessional Residency Program in Physical Rehabilitation, tutor at the Residency Program in Cancer Care and at the Residency Program in Children's Health, and responsible for the implementation, technical assistance and teaching in the public health service of the first and only Hypermobility and Ehlers-Danlos Syndromes Outpatient Clinic in Brazil. Dr. Neuseli Lamari was the owner of the Lamari Physiotherapy Clinic in the city of São José do Rio Preto, which she founded in 1982.

The biggest highlight in Dr. Neuseli's life has been being a mother of two children, who are her great companions. Her son, Mateus, is a Physiotherapist and a University Professor with a Master's degree and a Ph.D. in joint hypermobility. Mateus is dedicated to teaching and research and patient care. He is also a preceptor in In-Service Teaching at the Hospital de Base of the Faculty of Medicine of São José do Rio Preto. Her daughter, Mariana Lamari, studied law and advises her mother and brother in almost everything.

References

Cavenaghi S, Carvalho-Marino LH, Oliveira PP, Lamari NM. Hipermobilidade articular em pacientes com prolapso da valva mitral. Arq Bras Cardiol (Impresso). 2009;93:307–311.

Cavenaghi S, Folchine AER, Marino LHC, Lamari NM. Prevalência de hipermobilidade articular e sintomas álgicos em trabalhadores industriais. Arquivos de Ciências da Saúde (FAMERP). 2006;13:66–70.

Lamari MM, Lamari NM, Araujo-Filho GM, Medeiros MP, Marques VRP, Pavarino EC. Psychosocial and motor characteristics of patients with hypermobility. Frontiers in Psychiatry. 2022. Frontiers in Psychiatry. https://doi.org/10.3389/fpsyt.2021.787822. 2022 Mar;12:787822.

Lamari MM, Lamari NM, Medeiros MP Pavarino EC. Signos y Síntomas en niños y adolescentes con Hipermovilidad Articular: un estudio transversal cuantitativo observacional. Rev chil reumatol 2020;36(2):42–53.

Lamari NM et al. Autism spectrum disorder and Ehlers-Danlos syndrome—hypermobility type: a case report. Arch Health Sci. 2021;28(1) ago.

Lamari NM, Carvalho-Marino LH, Marino Junior NW, Cordeiro JA, Pellegrini AM. Flexão Anterior do Tronco no adolescente após o pico de velocidade de crescimento em estatura. Acta Ortop Bras 2007;15(1):25–9.

Lamari NM, Chueire AG, Cordeiro JA. Analysis of joint mobility patterns among preschool children. São Paulo Med J 2005;123(3):119–23.

Lamari NM, Cordeiro JA, Carvalho-Marino LHC. Intervening factors in forward flexibility of the trunk in adolescents in sitting and standing position. Minerva Pediatr: a journal on pediatrics, neonatology, adolescent medicine, child and adolescent psychiatry. 2010;62:353–361.

Lamari NM, Lamari MM, Medeiros MP. Systemic Manifestations of Ehlers-Danlos Syndrome Hypermobility Type. MOJ Cell Sci. 2017;4.

Lamari NM, Lamari MM. Characterization of Brazilian children with joint hypermobility. Int J Physiatry. 2016;2:011.

Lamari NM, Marino LHC, Marino Junior NW, Cordeiro JA. Estudo da Mobilidade Articular Generalizada e índices de Flexibilidade Anterior do Tronco na Comunidade Japonesa em Guaíra e São José do Rio Preto. HB Científica (FUNFARME). 2003 São José do Rio Preto-SP, 10(2):73–83.

Marino LHC, Lamari NM, Marino Junior NW. Hipermobilidade articular nos joelhos da criança. Arquivos de Ciências da Saúde (FAMERP), São José do Rio Preto-SP, v. 11, p. 124–127, 2004.

Miller SMC, Lamari MM, Lamari NM. Síndrome de Ehlers-Danlos Tipo Hipermobilidade: Estratégias de Inclusão. Arq Cien Saúde. 2015; Síndrome de Ehlers-Danlos tipo hipermobilidade: estratégias de inclusão. Arq. Ciênc. Saúde. 2015;22(1):21–27. http://lattes.cnpq.br/8155176727053805

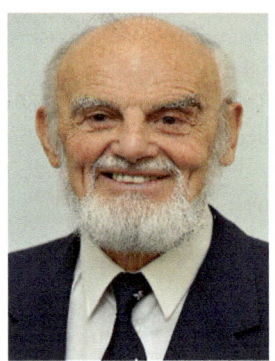

Dr. Peter Beighton (Medical Geneticist) OMB, M.D., Ph.D., FRCP, FRS (SA), FRS (UK) was the first recipient of the newly established Order of Mapungubwe (bronze), 2002, which was bestowed by the South African President, Mbeki. He was followed on the podium by former Presidents de Klerk and Mandela, who received the award in gold and platinum, respectively. Dr. Beighton's Award reflected his lifetime achievement as a scientist and for his research into inherited medical disorders in South Africa.

Dr. Beighton was born in Lancashire, England in 1934 and qualified in medicine in 1957 at St. Mary's Hospital, University of London. After several internships in this hospital group, he served as a Medical Officer in the Parachute Regiment and with the United Nations forces during the Congo Crisis. In 1966, he trained in internal medicine at St. Thomas's Hospital in London and wrote a Doctoral Thesis on the Ehlers-Danlos Syndrome. He later held a Fulbright Fellowship in Clinical Genetics in 1968–1969 with Dr. Victor McKusick at Johns Hopkins Hospital in Baltimore, USA.

In 1968, Beighton published a report in the *British Heart Journal* stating that air travel can produce 'an ideal climate for precipitating deep vein thrombosis' (1968). This report was not taken seriously and passengers were not warned about the possible dangers. It was only in the early 1990s that the link between long flights and deep vein thrombosis was made public. His report had been based on his experience at Hillingdon Hospital, West London, where air travellers with acute medical problems were regularly admitted from London Airport.

During the 1960s, and in between hospital appointments in London, Beighton undertook clinical research during exploration expeditions in the Sahara Desert. He also carried out epidemiologic studies on Easter Island and Tristan da Cunha.

In 1970, Beighton and his newly-wed wife, Greta, spent a year based in the Division of Orthopaedic Surgery, University of Witwatersrand, Johannesburg. The purpose was to conduct large-scale epidemiological studies in indigenous populations of South Africa. This successful project resulted in a Ph.D. and formed the basis for current clinical assessment of an individual's range of joint movements, which is known as the "Beighton Score".

It is relevant that Greta made major contributions to the conception and implementation of the "Score" and it is entirely appropriate they she should share the eponymous recognition that is usually accorded to Peter. It is of interest that their discussion, which led to this formulation, was held around a campfire in the Kalahari Desert.

In 1972, Beighton was appointed Professor of Human Genetics at the University of Cape Town's Faculty of Medicine. A sabbatical at the University of Cambridge was facilitated in 1979 by an Oppenheimer Fellowship. In addition to his Departmental duties at the University of Cape Town, he was also appointed as Director of an MRC Unit for Medical Genetics. His research was largely on inherited disorders of the skeleton and connective tissues and also involved genetic conditions which cause deafness, physical disability and visual problems. Much of the research was undertaken at special schools for children with these conditions. Over the years, these facilities were visited by Beighton and his team and several thousand affected children were examined and documented across South Africa. Genetic counselling for the children and their parents was an inherent component of this process.

Dr. Beighton has received several awards, including the Gold Medal of the British Orthopaedic Association (1975), the President's Medallion of the South African Orthopaedic Association (1978), the Smith & Nephew Literary Award (1979) and the Silver Medal of the South African Medical Research Council (1997). In 2002, he was the first recipient of the South African Order of Mapungubwe (Bronze).

He is a Fellow of the Royal Colleges of Physicians of Edinburgh (1975) and London (1978). In the period 1970–1990, he was also accorded Fellowships of the University of Cape Town, the British Society of Rheumatology and the Royal Geographical Society. In this period, he was Vice-President of the Royal Society of South Africa and Chairman of the South African Human Genetics Society.

In 1999, at the age of 65, Beighton obtained the degree of Master of Philosophy in Social History by external thesis at the University of Lancaster, UK. This thesis was entitled *Blackpool Division, St. John Ambulance Brigade: The Early Years*. Professor Beighton reached obligatory retirement age at the end of 1999 and was accorded the status of Emeritus Professor in Human Genetics. He retained his links with UCT and continued his long-standing collaboration with the Faculty of Dentistry at the University of the Western Cape. He was the subject of a Festschrift published as a supplement to the *South African Medical Journal* on 1 June 2016, which honoured his knowledge, leadership and mentorship in the field of medical genetics.

Over the years, 16 of his post-graduate students were awarded Ph.Ds., including three from the Dental Faculty, UWC. The last of these students received this distinction at UCT in April 2019. Ten of the 16 Ph.D. students achieved Associate or Full Professorial status in universities around the world. Fourteen of Professor Beighton's postgraduate students have been awarded Doctorates and nine of them have achieved Professorial status. Professor Beighton is the author, co-author or editor of 20 monographs and editions, 34 chapters and more than 440 medical publications.

Professor Beighton and his wife, Greta, a multi-talented nursing sister whom he met in 1958 at Paddington General Hospital in London, travelled widely and undertook extensive collaborative medical research together. They also shared an interest in the history of medical genetics and jointly authored two unique volumes of brief biographies of people for whom genetic syndromes have been named.

Sporting activities were continued throughout Beighton's life. He played rugby at St. Mary's Hospital as a medical student and enjoyed his last game there at the age of 50, while passing through London on Professorial duties. In Cape Town, he took up running and participated in numerous conventional and off-road events, including the Two Oceans and Comrades Marathons. In his mid-seventies, he became involved in cycle racing in the Cape and was aided and encouraged by his beloved wife, Greta, until her final illness put an end to these activities in 2014. Sadly, Greta died in Cape Town on 29 May 2017.

In the empty years that followed, Peter remained in the family home in Cape Town. His writing activities continued and in 2022 at the age of 88 years, this brief biographical summary was finally completed.

References

Beighton P, Beighton G. The man behind the syndrome. Springer; 1986. p 240.

Beighton P, Beighton G. The person behind the syndrome. Springer; 1996. p 231.

Beighton P, de Paepe A, Danks D, Finidori G, Gedde-Dahl T, Goodman R, et al. International nosology of heritable disorders of connective tissue, Berlin, 1986. Am J Med Genet. 1988.

Beighton P, de Paepe A, Danks D, Finidori G, Gedde-Dahl T, Goodman R, et al. International nosology of heritable disorders of connective tissue, Berlin, 1986. Am J Med Genet. 1988;29:581–94.

Beighton P, De Paepe A, Steinmann B, Tsipouras P, Wenstrup RJ. Ehlers-Danlos syndromes: revised nosology, Villefranche, 1997. Ehlers-Danlos National Foundation (USA) and Ehlers-Danlos Support Group (UK). Am J Med Genet. 1998;77:31–7.

Beighton P, ed. McKusick's. Heritable disorders of connective tissue. 5th ed. St. Louis: Mosby; 1993.

Beighton P, Grahame R, Bird H. Hymobility of joints. Springer; 1983. p 178.

Beighton P, Grahame R, Bird HA. Hypermobility of joints, 4th ed. London, UK: Springer; 2012. p 204.

Beighton P, Murdoch JL, Votteler T. Gastrointestinal complication of the Ehlers-Danlos syndrome. Gut 1969;10:1004–1008.

Beighton P, Solomon I, Soskolne L. Articular mobility in an African population. Ann Rheum Dis. 1973;32:413–8.

Beighton P. The Ehlers-Danlos syndrome. London: William Heinemann Medical Books; 1970.

Beighton PH, Horan FT. Dominant inheritance in familial generalised articular hypermobility. J Bone Joint Surg Br. 1970;52:145–7.

1

Contributors to the Understanding of the EDS and Hypermobility in Antiquity

Introduction

Current concepts are based upon early case reports concerning the Elhers-Danlos Syndrome in which an excessive range of joint movements is a major diagnostic feature (Littré and Bailliere 1840). Brief biographical and syndromic information is presented in chronological order of the individual publications in the field of hypermobility.

In his writings "Airs, Waters and Places", Hippocrates stated that the Scythian nomads inhabiting the region that currently forms part of the Ukraine and Slovakia (Crimea) often had loose joints and multiple scars. Their "elastic" shoulders and loose elbows make them incapable of drawing bowstrings or throwing spears with the same skill as their enemies, who could hurl their weapons up to 500 m. Equally, this condition enabled them to be skilled horsemen, since they could wrap their legs and feet around the

© The Author(s), under exclusive license to Springer Nature Switzerland AG 2023
N. Lamari and P. Beighton, *Hypermobility in Medical Practice*,
In Clinical Practice, https://doi.org/10.1007/978-3-031-34914-0_1

belly of a horse with an ability that their enemies lacked. At the time, it was believed that their scars had been caused by cauterisations applied in an attempt to stiffen the joints (Littré and Bailliere 1840; Asociación Síndromes de Ehlers-Danlos e Hiperlaxitud 2017).

Jorge Albes was a 23-year-old Spanish patient who presented at the Leyden Academy in Amsterdam in 1657 by Dutch surgeon Job Janszoon van Meek'ren (Littré and Bailliere 1840; Steinmann et al. 2002; Easton et al. 2014; Malfait and Paepe 2014; Hamonet et al. 2016; Asociación Síndromes de Ehlers-Danlos e Hiperlaxitud 2017). Albes could stretch the skin of his right shoulder with his left hand up to his mouth. He could also cover his face with the skin from his chin and stretch it to his chest. Job van Meek'ren is believed to have made the first partial description of the manifestations of hypermobility (Steinmann et al. 2002; Malfait and Paepe 2014; Hamonet et al. 2016).

Peter Rubens depicted hyperextension of the metacarpal joints, hyperflexion of the feet and hyperlordosis in his work "*The Three Graces*" (1638–1640), which is hanging in the *Museo del Prado* in Madrid (Dequeker 2001). The musical success of Paganini at the turn of the 19th Century was attributed to the extreme mobility of his hands (Larsson et al. 1993; Cherpel and Marks 1999; Simmonds and Keer 2007).

In 1891, the Russian dermatologist Alexander Nikolayev Tschernogobow presented two patients at the Dermatology and Venereology Society in Moscow. The first, a 17-year-old, had repeated articular luxations with frail hyperextensible skin, multiple scars as the result of minor trauma, difficulty healing and molluscoid pseudotumours on the knees, elbows and other parts of the body. Tschernogobow attributed these lesions to a disease of the connective tissue. The second of his patients was a

57-year-old man who had undergone operations for various tumours and experienced severe problems with the resultant scars (Parapia and Jackson 2008; Hamonet et al. 2016).

In the book "*Anomalies and Curiosities of Medicine*", Gould and Pyle (1897) mention a man from Budapest, who appeared in circus sideshows under the name "Elastic-Skin Man". He exhibited accentuated stretching of the skin of his entire body together with an "elastic" nose. These authors also reproduced a photograph of an exhibitionist named Felix Wehrle, who could not only stretch his skin, but could easily bend his fingers back to an extreme position.

Edvard Ehlers, Dermatologist (1863–1937)

Edvard Ehlers was an eminent Danish dermatologist at the turn of the century. He was born in Copenhagen, Denmark in 1863. His father was the mayor of the city and he spent his childhood in comfortable circumstances. After a classical education Ehlers qualified in medicine in 1891. Early in his career, he developed an interest in dermatology and wrote a thesis entitled "*Extirpation of the Primary Lesion of Syphilis*". Thereafter, he undertook postgraduate studies in Berlin, Breslau, Vienna and Paris, before returning to practice in Copenhagen.

Ehlers was appointed chief of the Dermatological Polyclinic at the Fredericks Hospital in 1906 and he was Director of the special service of the Commune Hospital in Copenhagen from 1911 until his retirement in 1932. He was also involved in the establishment of the Welander Asylum for individuals with congenital syphilis, where he placed great emphasis on rehabilitation and specific treatment. Ehlers received numerous academic honours and became president of the International Union Against Venereal Disease.

In his prime, Ehlers was a tall man with fair hair and blue eyes, gold-rimmed spectacles, intellectual charm and a distinguished bearing. He was an indefatigable traveller and spoke several languages. Ehlers had a talent for organisation and was involved in projects concerning leprosy control and prevention in the West Indies and Iceland, syphiloid on Jutland and Mal de Meleda (inherited symmetrieal keratodermia of the extremities) on an island off the coast of Dalmatia.

Ehlers was frequently present at international congresses and gained a reputation as a witty toastmaster and after-dinner speaker on these occasions. His travels often took him to France where he was a regular participant in the clinical meetings of the French Dermatological Society. Paris was his favourite city and he knew and enjoyed many facets of the Parisian way of life; of his three wives, the first was French. During the First World War, Ehlers organised a field ambulance service and directed the evacuation of wounded French servicemen to Denmark. He died in 1937, at the age of 74, after a brief but painful illness.

In 1899, Ehlers presented a 21-year-old law student from Bornholm Island at a clinical meeting and the case report was later published in the dermatological literature. This patient had delayed walking and frequent subluxations of the knees. He also had many haematomata on minor trauma, with the formation of discoloured lesions on the elbows, knees and knuckles. In addition, he had extensible skin and lax digits.

Ehlers was a proponent of diagnostic humility, but he equally recognised the importance of syndromic delineation. At the beginning of this case presentation, he stated

"It is never difficult for me, whether faced by colleagues or patients, to admit that I know nothing about a given case, and I always wonder about colleagues who insist on fastening a label on every disorder. It is much more important to classify, mark and define diseases on the basis of aetiology than to label them as isolated, rare and hitherto unobserved cases."

The parents and three sisters of Ehlers's patient were considered normal. In view of present-day concepts, the question arises as to whether the young man represented a new mutation for the common autosomal dominant form of the disease or whether he had a rare disease autosomal recessive or X-linked type. It would be of great academic interest to know if there are any affected descendants on Bornholm Island or elsewhere in Scandinavia.

Danlos presented a similar case to the Dermatological Society of Paris in 1908 and three decades later the conjoined eponym gained general acceptance. The condition has been the subject of extensive reviews and more than a thousand cases have now been reported. Current interest is centred upon the recognition of heterogeneity and the definition of the basic defect at biochemical and molecular levels.

Material in this brief account of Ehlers was previously published in a monograph "The Man Behind the Syndrome." ed. Beighton G and Beighton P. Springer-Verlag 1986.

Henri-Alexandre Danlos, Dermatologist (1844–1912)

Henri-Alexandre Danlos was born in Paris on 26 March 1844 and his whole life was spent in that city and he was a French physician, an innovator in the field of dermatological therapeutics.

He qualified in Medicine with a distinction in 1869 and in 1874 presented his doctoral thesis, which was entitled *The Relationship between Menstruation and Skin Disease.* Danlos retained an early interest in chemistry and undertook research at the Wurtz Laboratory in this phase of his career. In 1881, at the age of 37, he passed an examination for the Consultant status *(médecin des hôpitaux).* Thereafter, he spent 5 years at the Hôpital Tenon, followed by 5 years in the public health service. This was an unhappy period for Danlos as he suffered a prolonged and painful illness, becoming withdrawn and pessimistic.

Danlos achieved his life's ambition in 1895 at the age of 51, when he was appointed to the Hôpital Saint Louis in Paris. He gained a reputation as a caring physician and excellent teacher, and he was increasingly involved in the development of new therapeutic techniques in dermatology. In the period 1895–1912, Danlos and undertook numerous meticulous studies of the use of various preparations of arsenic and mercurials in the treatment of syphilis and other skin disorders. He also carried out pioneering investigations of the role of radium and X-rays in dermatology and published several papers on these topics.

Danlos's scientific work received recognition in 1904 when he was elected as president of the Paris Medical Society. In 1906, he became the secretary of the Dermatological Society of Paris. Despite these successes he continued to be depressed and for many years was never seen to smile. He had an abrupt manner but nevertheless retained the affection and sympathy of his colleagues. His health issues persisted, and he died on 12 September 1912 at the age of 68 in his home in Chatou.

In 1908, Danlos discussed a patient at the Paris Society of Dermatology and Syphilology. This boy had lesions on his elbows and knees and had been presented to the same Society 18 months earlier by Danlos's colleagues, Hallopeau and Macé de Lépinay, with the diagnosis of juvenile pseudo-xanthomata. Danlos disagreed with this diagnosis and drew attention to the extensibility and fragility of the patient's skin and to his propensity for bruising. He gave a detailed analysis of his reasons for believing that the lesions over the bony prominences were post-traumatic "pseudo-tumours" in a patient with an inherent defect which he termed "cutis laxa". In the ensuing discussion, Hallopeau maintained that his original diagnosis was correct. Danlos, with characteristic firmness, negated his argument and played his trump card by mentioning that similar cases had been reported in Denmark by Ehlers in 1901 and at the Berne congress by Kohn in 1906.

The first complete case description of the condition, which became known as the Ehlers-Danlos syndrome, was given by Tschernogobow in 1892 when he presented two patients at the Moscow Dermatological and Venereologic Society. The disorder still carries his eponym in Russia. In hindsight, the syndrome can also be diagnosed in a Spaniard who was presented by the Dutch surgeon, van Meekren, at the Academy of Leyden in 1657.

Isolated case reports continued to appear during the early part of the twentieth century under a variety of designations and semantic confusion developed. Parkes Weber resolved these difficulties in 1936, shortly before Ehlers's death, when he pointed out that dermal extensibility and fragility, in association with articular laxity and molluscoid pseudo-tumours, had been features of the original patients. Weber's proposal that the condition should be termed "Ehlers-Danlos syndrome" has gained universal acceptance.

Frederick Parkes Weber, Physician (1863–1962)

Frederick Parkes Weber was an eminent physician in London during the first half of the twentieth century. He had a lifelong interest in rare disorders and for many years he was the doyen of British syndromic diagnosticians. He was born in 1863 and educated at Charterhouse School, Cambridge University and St. Bartholomew's Hospital, London. His father, Sir Hermann Weber, came to England from Germany as a young man and became Queen Victoria's physician.

Weber derived his middle name "Parkes" from his father's great friend, Sir Edmund Parkes and in time this forename became coupled with his surname, so that he was generally known as "Parkes Weber". His family retained their Germanic connections and Weber pronounced his surname in the continental "V" manner.

After qualification, Weber held resident posts at Bart's and Brompton Hospital before being appointed as honorary physician to the German Hospital, Queen Square, London, in 1894. In this capacity, he carried on with his duties until he reached his 80th year.

Weber remained active at the Royal Society of Medicine until after the age of 90 and he was frequently called upon to resolve difficult diagnostic dilemmas by virtue of his legendary knowledge of rare disorders. It is recorded in his obituary that when, for the first time in his life, he stated at a meeting of the Society that he had "never heard of the syndrome" that was under discussion, tumultuous applause broke out, followed by cheers and stamping of feet; the noise reached a crescendo and the meeting was abandoned in disorder!

Weber was noted for the clarity of his diction and for the quality of his prolific publications. Over a span of 50 years, he wrote over 1200 medical articles and contributed to more than 20 books or chapters. Many of these reports concerned new entities and for this reason his name has been attached to several unusual disorders. Weber was especially interested in dermatological conditions and shortly before his death he founded a prize at the Royal College of Physicians to promote this speciality; this award is bestowed in conjunction with a lecture which bears his name.

Weber was meticulous in his approach to clinical problems and unfailingly courteous to patients and colleagues. He achieved contentment and success in all facets of his life and was universally liked and respected. In turn, he liked everybody and was interested in everything. Weber was an avid collector of coins, medals and antiques and was a member of several learned societies relating to these pursuits.

In 1918, Weber added the additional component of arteriovenous fistulae and, thereafter, the triple eponym came into use. Confusion arose and various combinations of the compound eponym were used for different groupings of these abnormalities. However, these diverse forms of the disorder are now usually lumped together under the term "KIippel-Trenaunay-Weber" syndrome. Weber's name is associated with at least six other disorders, of which the Osler-Rendu-Weber and Sturge-Weber syndromes are the best known. It is less well known that in 1936 Weber was the originator of the eponym "Ehlers-Danlos Syndrome".

Weber became blind and deaf during old age and passed his final years in his flat in Harley Street. He retained his intellectual faculties until the end and died peacefully in 1962 in his 100th year.

References

Asociación Síndromes de Ehlers-Danlos e Hiperlaxitud. Ehlers Danlos. Disponível em: https://ehlersdanlos.org.es/sin-drome-de-hiperlaxitud-articular. Acessado em: 29 July 2017.

Cherpel A, Marks R. The benign joint hypermobility syndrome. N Z J Physiother. 1999;27:9–22.

Dequeker J. Benign familial hypermobility syndrome and Trendelenburg sign in a painting "The Three Graces" by Peter Paul Rubens (1577–1640). Ann Rheum Dis. 2001;60:894–989.

Easton V, Bale P, Bacon H, Jerman E, Armon K, Macgregor AJ. A89: the relationship between Benign joint hypermobility syndrome and developmental coordination disorders in children. Arthritis Rheum. 2014;66(Suppl 3):S124.

Gould GM, Pyle WL. Anomalies and curiosities of medicine. London: Rebman; 1897.

Hamonet C, Ducret L, Layadi K, Baeza C. Historia y actualidad del Síndrome de Ehlers-Danlos-Tschernogobow. Cuad Neuropsicol. 2016;10:17–31.

Larsson LG, Baum J, Mudholkar GS, Kollia GD. Benefits and disadvantages of joint hypermobility among musicians. N Engl J Med. 1993;329:1079–82.

Littré E, Bailliere JB. Oeuvres complètes d'Hippocrate. Paris: La Bibliothèque Interuniversitaire de Médecine de Paris; 1840.

Malfait F, De Paepe A. The Ehlers-Danlos syndrome. Adv Exp Med Biol. 2014;802:129–43.

Parapia LA, Jackson C. Ehlers-Danlos syndrome-a historical review. Br J Haematol. 2008;141:32–5.

Simmonds JV, Keer R. Hypermobility and the hypermobility syndrome. Man Ther. 2007;12:298–309.

Steinmann B, Royce PM, Superti-Furga A. The Ehlers-Danlos syndrome. In: Royce PM, Steinmann B, editors. Connective tissue and its heritable disorders: molecular, genetic, and medical aspects. 2nd ed. Hoboken: Wiley; 2002. p. 687–725.

Ehlers

Beighton P. The Ehlers-Danlos syndrome. London: William Heinemann; 1970.

Danlos H. Un cas de cutis laxa avec tumeurs par contusion chronique des coudes et des genoux. Bull Soc Fr Derm Syph. 1908a;19:70.

Ehlers E. Cutis laxa, Neigung zu Haemorrhagien in der Haut, Lockerung mehrerer Artikulationen (case for diagnosis). Derm Z. 1901;8:173.

McKusick VA. Heritable disorders of connective tissue, 4th ed. St. Louis: CV Mosby; 1973. p. 292–371.

Danlos

Danlos H. Un cas de cutis laxa avec tumeurs par contusion chronique des coudes et des genoux (xanthome juvenile pseudodiabetique de MM Hallopeau et Macé de Lepinay). Bull Soe Fr Derm Syph. 1908b;19:70.

Denko CW. Chernogubov's syndrome: a translation of the first modern case report of the Ehlers-Danlos syndrome. J Rheumatol. 1978;5:347.

Obituary (1912) *Bull Soc Derm Syph*, Paris. p. 500.

Weber FP. The Ehlers-Danlos syndrome. Hr J Dermatol Syph. 1936a;48:609.

Weber

Klippel M, Trenaunay R. Du naevus variqueux osteohypertrophique. Arch Gen Med. 1900;185:641.

McKusick VA. Frederick Parkes Weber, 1863–1962. JAMA. 1963;183:131.

Obituary. Lancet I; 1962, p. 1308.

Weber FP. Angioma formation in connection with hypertrophy of limbs and hemihypertrophy. Br J Dermatol. 1907;19:231.

Weber FP. Haemangiectatic hypertrophy of limbs congenital phlebarteriectasis and so-called varicose veins. Br J Child Dis. 1918;15:13.

Weber FP. Ehlers-Danlos syndrome. Proc R Soc Med. 1936b;30:1.

2

Contributors to the Understanding of Hypermobility and Ehlers-Danlos Syndrome in the Modern Era

Introduction

In the early 1950's, after the chaos of WWII had subsided, interest in familial disorders began to expand in both pediatric and adult medicine. This process lead to the development of Medical Genetics as a research interest and subsequently evolved into an accepted medical speciality with the establishment of consultant posts at major academic hospitals in the UK, USA and continental Europe. As in the previous sections, brief biographical information concerning the major contributors to the understanding of Hypermobility is presented in this chapter. The author, PB was acquainted with most of them and they were regarded as personal friends.

Joint hypermobility or articular hyperlaxity is conventually defined by the Beighton score (Beighton et al. 1973). This index is commonly used and perhaps the most reliable professional tool for evaluating GJH (Juul-Kristensen

© The Author(s), under exclusive license to Springer Nature Switzerland AG 2023
N. Lamari and P. Beighton, *Hypermobility in Medical Practice*, In Clinical Practice, https://doi.org/10.1007/978-3-031-34914-0_2

et al. 2007). In an extensive review on JH, the concept of hypermobility spectrum disorders (HSDs) was created (Castori et al. 2017). In this approach, the continuity of JH, asymptomatic or symptomatic, as well as to documentation of its location, age group and natural history can be recognised. The authors proposed that individuals with JH can be classified as follows:

1. Asymptomatic and non-syndromic persons with JH;
2. Individuals with JH who meet the criteria for Hypermobile form of the Ehlers-Danlos syndrome (hEDS).
3. Symptomatic persons with JH who do not meet the diagnostic criteria for hEDS are regarded as having HSDs.

Cedric Carter, Geneticist (1917–1984)

Professor Cedric Carter was director of the Medical Research Council's Clinical Genetics Unit at the Institute of Child Health, London until his retirement in 1982. He established the Clinical Genetics Society in 1970 and as its first president he provided guidance in the early years. On his retirement, the Society honoured his contribution to clinical genetics by establishing The Carter Lecture, the first of which was given in 1984.

Cedric Carter was a private, modest person, greatly loved by those who worked with him. He had an enormous influence on the development of clinical genetics. Not only did he train many of those now practicing or teaching clinical genetics in Britain, he was also largely responsible for setting up a network of genetic clinics and centres with consultant posts. He was also responsible for the official recognition of clinical genetics as a separate specialty in the NHS. His influence extended abroad, and he helped to establish clinical genetics in many parts of the world.

Cedric Carter developed his interests as research fellow in congenital malformations at the Hospital for Sick Children, Great Ormond Street in 1948. In 1952, as part time research fellow in genetics, he joined Dr. Fraser Roberts when he started the genetic clinic at that hospital. He also became a member of the scientific staff of the Medical Research Council's Genetic Unit when it was established in the Institute of Child Health in 1957.

He was appointed as a Consultant Geneticist at the Hospital for Sick Children in 1958 and at Queen Charlotte's Hospital in 1973. In 1964, he took over from Dr. Fraser Roberts as director of the MRC unit. He was also the consultant advisor in genetics to the Department of Health and Social Security from 1972 and professor of clinical genetics in the University of London from 1975 until his retirement.

Professor Carter's major scientific contributions concerned the common congenital malformations: not only did he contribute greatly to the understanding of genetic mechanisms but he also provided the data on which genetic counselling is now based. His meticulous family studies, usually based on a consecutive series of cases presenting at the Hospital for Sick Children, provided reliable data on the incidence of the disorder in first, second and third degree relatives. This process also allowed him to consolidate the concept of multifactorial inheritance as applied to congenital malformations.

He wrote over 70 papers reporting original work, over 100 review articles, more than 30 chapters in books, and 3 complete books. Cedric Carter died in 1984 at the age of 67 years.

Victor A. Mckusick, Medical Geneticist (1921–2008)

Victor McKusick was Emeritus Professor of Pediatrics and Medical Genetics at UBC & Center for Children's and Women's Health, British Columbia, Canada. He was a world figure and ranks as the founder of Medical Genetics. Victor Almon McKusick was born October 21, 1921 in Parkman, Maine, USA and died at the age of 86 years on July 22, 2008 in Baltimore, USA.

He attended Tufts College and then entered the Johns Hopkins Hospital Medical School. He developed an interest in internal medicine, then cardiology, and finally in human/medical genetics. Thereafter he received a prestigious Fellowship to stay and work at the Johns Hopkins Hospital. Dr. McKusick trained more than 300 Fellows and he was the forerunner of today's medical genetic training programs in the USA.

During his lifetime, medical genetics went from an esoteric, backwater subject to the very essence of modern biology and medicine. Dr. McKusick was at the forefront of that whole process. He emphasized the role of genetics in many human disorders and, through OMIM, made the appropriate references widely available. He was also instrumental in the development of the Human Genome Project.

He contributed to committees and policy making, maintained OMIM entries, and responded to new developments over many years. He was somewhat shy but had always a patient's best interest at heart. With a long-term interest in the genetics of short stature, he was made an honorary member of the Little People of America (LPA). Dr. McKusick has received many honors and awards and he had 21 honorary degrees.

McKusick was a member of the National Academy of Sciences, the Institute of Medicine and the American Philosophical Society. He received many awards including the National Medal of Science (the highest scientific honor in the US). He was President of the American Society of Human Genetics and HUGO (Human Genome Organization), the Editor of the journal Genomics and Medicine, the primary contributor to MIM (Mendelian Inheritance in Man), and subsequently to the online version OMIM (which now has over 18,000 entries).

Dr. McKusick worked for more than 60 years at the Johns Hopkins Hospital School of Medicine. He was active until the last week of his life. Victor McKusick died in 2008.

Howard Bird. Rheumatogist (1940?–2021)

Howard Bird was an emeritus Professor of Pharmacological Rheumatology at the University of Leeds following his retirement in 2010 from the posts of Academic Sub-Dean and Honorary Consultant Rheumatologist. As a clinician, he was responsible for the Leeds Rheumatology Clinic which was devoted to Inherited Abnormalities of Connective Tissue.

His MD thesis was entitled 'Joint Hypermobility' and he wrote numerous books, chapters and original scientific articles. He took an interest in loose joints from the Rheumatological standpoint in the 1960's and was a co-author of Peter Beighton's book "Hypermobility of Joints", which went into several editions.

In 2011, Bird was appointed as Visiting Professor at University College London in conjunction with their newly established Msc in Performing Arts Medicine. He had held clinics for musicians and dancers for nearly 20 years. In this context he was a teacher and scientific researcher in Performing Arts Medicine and in Joint Flexibility at University College, the Laban Conservatoire for Dance and at the Royal College of Music. Howard Bird died in 2021.

Frank Horan, Orthopaedic Surgeon (1933–2015)

Frank Horan was a renowned orthopaedic surgeon specialising in sports medicine. In cricket; he was a medical adviser to Lord's and MCC and for 30 years he oversaw the treatment of English and foreign players during test matches and county fixtures. Horan died at the age of 82.

Francis Thomas Horan was born in Manchester on July 24 in 1933 and educated at Torquay Grammar School, where his passions were cricket, cycling and table tennis. In 1951, he won a place to study Medicine at St Mary's Hospital, Paddington, but failed his first-year exams and was expelled. Obligatory National Service in the RAF followed and he was a radar operator for Fighter Control while studying to retake his exams. Having passed these in Dublin, he persuaded the Dean of St Mary's to re-admit him—a rare occurrence—and qualified in 1959.

A research fellowship in Montreal led to an MSc from McGill University in 1974 and on his return to the UK, Horan was appointed as a consultant Orthopaedic surgeon at the Cuckfield Hospital in Sussex, where he eventually became medical director.

His main area of academic interest was dysplasias (deformities) of the bones, and he published more than 20 papers on the subject. Many of these were co-authored with his lifelong friend Peter Beighton, a fellow student at St Mary's and later Professor of Genetics at the University of Cape Town. The dysplasias that interested them were linked to hereditary disorders such as some forms of dwarfism. In the early 1970s, the two men spent many months in South Africa flying to clinics in remote parts of the Transkei and KwaZulu Natal in search of unusual examples. A skeletal disorder which they discovered—Horan-Beighton Syndrome—carries their eponyms.

Horan had an affinity for the written word and cherished his appointment in 1998 as Editor of the Journal of Bone and Joint Surgery. In this context he edited and re-wrote hundreds of international submissions on developments in orthopaedics. He travelled to South America, the Far East and Australia promoting this publication and he lectured widely on how to present scientific papers.

He was a keen rugby player as a student and in later life during his regular visits to Cape Town he developed a taste for running, and ran the Peninsula marathon three times, allowing himself a cigarette at the end of a particularly demanding hill. In 1981, adopting a more orthodox smoke-free approach, he completed the inaugural London marathon in 3 h 59 min.

In 1962, Frank Horan was married to Cynthia Bambury, who was a nurse at St Mary's Hospital at the time. She and their daughter and two sons survive him. Frank Horan, born July 24, 1933, died in 2015.

Rodney Grahame, Rheumatologist (1932–)

Rodney Grahame graduated in 1965 from the London Hospital Medical College (University of London) and has been in continuous medical practice for 60 years.

Formerly, he was a consultant rheumatologist at Guy's Hospital and University College London Trust and a former paediatric rheumatologist Gt. Ormond Street Hospital for Children. He is also an Honorary Professor at the Division of Medicine, University College London and Affiliate Professor, in the Department of Pathology, School of Medicine, University of Washington, Seeatle WA, USA. His awards are: CBE, Queen's Birthday Award for services to Rheumatology and Disability Living Allowance Advisory Board 1998; Ehlers-Danlos Syndrome Society Life-time Achievement Award 2016; Elected to the Mastership, American College of Rheumatology 2017.

Rodney Grahame was appointed as a consultant in rheumatology and rehabilitation at Guy's Hospital in London in 1969. This position he held until 1997 when he moved to University College London Hospitals as emeritus professor and part/time consultant rheumatologist. He is a former editor of 'Rheumatology' and has held the Presidency of the British Society for Rheumatology, the British League against Rheumatism (now renamed ARMA), and the Section of Rheumatology & Rehabilitation of the Royal Society of Medicine. From 1987 to 1995 he was Chairman of the Education and Publications Committee of the International League of Associations of Rheumatology (ILAR).

In 1990, the University of London conferred the title of Professor of Clinical Rheumatology. He was also elected to the fellowships of the Royal College of Physicians of London, the American College of Physicians, the British Society for Rheumatology and the Royal Society of Arts. In 1998, he was awarded the title of Commander of the Order of the British Empire (CBE) and he was also honoured by the national rheumatology societies of France, Russia and the Czech Republic. He is an advisor to the Hypermobility Syndrome Association (HMSA).

In 2004 Grahame was appointed as an Honorary Consultant in Paediatric Rheumatology at the Great Ormond Street Hospital for Children in London and Honorary Professor at University College London in the Department of Medicine. In 2010, he was appointed Afilliate Professor in the Department of Pathology, University of Washington.

Rodney Grahame is the author of almost 200 publications on the Joint Hypermobility Syndrome.

Alan E. H. Emery (1928–), Medical Geneticist

Alan Emery was an outstanding international figure in Medical Genetics and received several high honours during his career at the University of Edinburgh in Scotland.

Emery was born in 1928 in Oldham, an industrial town in Lancashire, UK, a few miles east of Manchester. He was quiet and unassuming during childhood but his considerable intellectual abilities were recognized at the local grammar school, where he was the top scholar. He then entered the University of Manchester and achieved a first class degree with distinction.

A two-year period of national service was obligatory in the UK for a few years after WWII and Emery was drafted into the army with the Kings Hussars.

He subsequently returned to Manchester University Medical School and qualified in medicine in 1960. His intellectual qualities had been retained and he was sent to the John Hopkins Hospital, USA where he was a research fellow with the great Victor McKusick. He obtained a PhD and became interested in human genetics. Thereafter he achieved eponymous immortality when his name was applied to a rare neuromuscular disorder which is widely known as the Emery-Dreifuss Syndrome. He is also widely remembered for his book "Elements of Medical Genetics" which was first published in the 1960s.

In 1968, at the age of 40 years, Emery was appointed as the Foundation Professor of Human Genetics at the University of Edinburgh. He then introduced a clinical service for patients with heritable disorders. This approach proved to be of considerable value in medical practice and by 2022 there were dedicated Genetic Counselling clinics. In this context, he is rightly regarded as the founder of Medical Genetics in the UK.

In 2022, Emery is alive and well at the age of 94 years. He still maintains his sense of humour and his interest in Medical Genetics.

References

Beighton P, Solomon I, Soskolne L. Articular mobility in an African population. Ann Rheum Dis. 1973;32:413–8.

Castori M, Tinkle B, Levy H, Grahame R, Malfait F, Hakim A. A framework for the classification of joint hypermobility and related conditions. Am J Med Genet C Semin Med Genet. 2017a;175:148–57.

Juul-Kristensen B, Røgind H, Jensen DV, Remvig L. Inter-examiner reproducibility of tests and criteria for generalized joint hypermobility and benign joint hypermobility syndrome. Rheumatology (Oxford). 2007;46:1835–41.

Carter

Carter C, Sweetnam R. Familial joint laxity and recurrent dislocation of the patella. J Bone Joint Surg Br. 1958;40-B:664–7.

Carter C, Sweetnam R. Recurrent dislocation of the patella and of the shoulder: their association with familial joint laxity. J Bone Joint Surg Br. 1960;42-B:721–727.

Carter C, Wilkinson LE. Persistent joint laxity and congenital dislocation of the hypermobility. J Bone Joint Surg Br. 1964;46B:40–5.

McKusick

Beighton P (ed). McKusick's heritable disorders of connective tissue. 5th ed. Mosby Baltimore, London, Sydney & Toronto; 1993.

McKusick VA. Heritable disorders of connective tissue. 4th ed. St.Louis: C. V. Mosby; 1972.

McKusick VA. Mendelian inheritance in man. 6th ed. Baltimore London: Johns Hopkins University Press; 1983.

Bird

Beighton P, Grahame R, Bird HA. Hypermobility of joints. 4th ed. London: Springer; 2012; vol 5. p. 65–94.

Bird HA. Overuse injuries in musicians. Br Med J. 1989;298:1129–30.

Bird HA. Joint hypermobility in children. Rheumatology (oxford). 2005;44(6):703–4.

Bird HA, Calguneri M. Joint mobility among university students. Br J Rheumatol. 1986;25:314.

Bird HA, Rathbone J, Nixon PGF. Over-use syndromes in musicians. Lancet. 1986;328:916–7.

Bird HA, Walker A, Newton J. A controlled study of joint laxity and injury in gymnasts. J Orthop Rheum. 1988;1:139–145.

Grahame R, Bird HA, Child A. The revised (Brighton 1998) criteria for the diagnosis of joint hypermobility syndrome (BJHS). J Rheumatol. 2000a;27:1777–9.

Tinkle BT, Bird HA, Grahame R, Lavallee M, Levy HP, Sillence D. The lack of clinical distinction between the hypermobility type of Ehlers-Danlos syndrome and the joint hypermobility syndrome (a.k.a. hypermobility syndrome). Am J Med Genet A. 2009;149A:2368–70.

Horan

Beighton P, Horan F. Orthopedic aspects of Ehlers-Danlos syndrome. J Bone Joint Surg Br. 1969;51(3):444–53.

Beighton PH, Horan FT. Dominant inheritance in familial generalised articular hypermobility. J Bone Joint Surg Br. 1970;52:145–7.

Horan FT, Beighton PH. Recessive inheritance of generalised articular hypermobility". Rheum Reahabil. 1973;12:47–49.

Obituary. The Times Newspaper. 2015.

Grahame

Beighton P, Grahame R, Bird HA. Hypermobility of joints, 4th ed. London: Springer; 2012;5:65–94.

Castori M, Tinkle B, Levy H, Grahame R, Malfait F, Hakim A. A framework for the classification of joint hypermobility and related conditions. Am J Med Genet C Semin Med Genet. 2017b;175:148–57.

Dolan AL, Hart DJ, Doyle DV, Grahame R, Spector TD. The relationship of joint hypermobility, bone mineral density, and osteoarthritis in the general population: the Chingford Study. J Rheumatol. 2003;30:799–803.

Grahame R. Joint hypermobility and the performing musician. N Engl J Med. 1993;329:1120–1.

Grahame R. Joint hypermobility and genetic collagen disorders: are they related? Arch Dis Child. 1999;80:188–91.

Grahame R. Ehlers-Danlos syndrome. S Afr Med J. 2016;106(6 Suppl 1):S45–6.

Grahame R, Beighton P. Physical properties of the skin in the Ehlers-Danlos syndrome. Ann Rheum Dis. 1969;28:246–52.

Grahame R, Jenkins JM. Joint hypermobility—asset or liability? a study of joint mobility in ballet dancers. Ann Rheum Dis. 1972;31:109–11.

Grahame R, Saunders AS, Maisey M. The use of scintigraphy in the diagnosis and management of traumatic foot lesions in ballet dancers. Rheumatology. 1979;18:235–8.

Grahame R, Edwards JC, Pitcher D, Gabell A, Harvey W. A clinical and echocardiographic study of patients with the hypermobility syndrome. Ann Rheum Dis. 1981;40:541–6.

Grahame R, Bird HA, Child A. The revised (Brighton 1998) criteria for the diagnosis of joint hypermobility syndrome (BJHS). J Rheumatol. 2000;27:1777–9.

Hakim AJ, Grahame R. A simple questionnaire to detect hypermobility: an adjunct to the assessment of patients with diffuse musculoskeletal pain. Int J Clin Pract. 2003;57:163–6.

Hakim AJ, Grahame R. Non-musculoskeletal symptoms in joint hypermobility syndrome. Indirect evidence for autonomic dysfunction? Rheumatology (Oxford) 2004;43:1194–5.

Tinkle BT, Bird HA, Grahame R, Lavallee M, Levy HP, Sillence D. The lack of clinical distinction between the hypermobility type of Ehlers-Danlos syndrome and the joint hypermobility syndrome (a.k.a. hypermobility syndrome). Am J Med Genet A. 2009;149A:2368–70.

Emery

Elements of Medical Genetics. Alan E.H. Emery. 1968.

Emery AE, Dreifuss FE. Unusual type of benign x-linked muscular dystrophy. J Neurol Neurosurg Psychiatry. 1966;29(4):338–42. https://doi.org/10.1136/jnnp.29.4.338. PMC1064196.PMID5969090.

Harper P, Reynolds L, Tansey T (eds). Clinical Genetics in Britain: origins and development. Wellcome Witnesses to Contemporary Medicine. History of Modern Biomedicine Research Group; 2010. ISBN 978-0-85484-127-1.

3

Assessment of the Magnitude of Joint Hypermobility

Introduction

Several methods have been developed for the assessment of the extent and severity of Generalised Joint Hypermobility (GJH). The first method was proposed by Carter and Wilkinson (1964), who considered five articular movements. This was followed in 1970 by a method proposed by Beighton and Horan (1970), using six articular movements in a family with autosomal dominant transmissionof GJH. Thereafter in 1973, Beighton et al. (1973) suggested an approach that considered five movements, scored from zero to nine points, with a score of 4 or more being indicative of GJH (Fig. 3.1).

In 2003, Hakim and Grahame (2003) developed a simple, reproducible self-report questionnaire as a tool to investigate JH retrospectively. This approach can be used to complement the clinical evaluation of chronic and diffuse pain syndromes where JH is sometimes not noticed.

© The Author(s), under exclusive license to Springer Nature Switzerland AG 2023
N. Lamari and P. Beighton, *Hypermobility in Medical Practice*, In Clinical Practice, https://doi.org/10.1007/978-3-031-34914-0_3

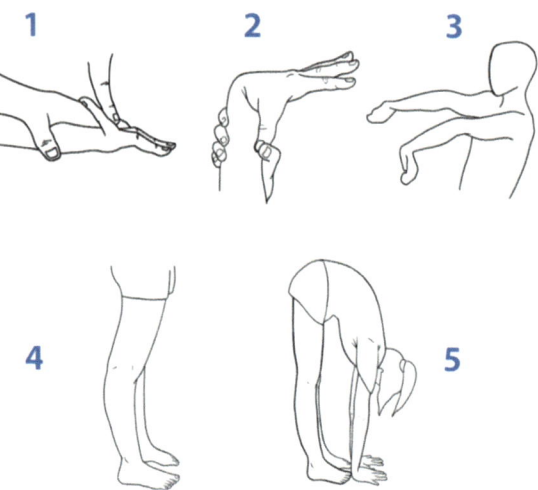

Fig. 3.1 Ilustration of Beighton's five variables for assessing generalized joint hypermobility (Mateus Lamari's doctoral thesis, 2021)

It is also applicable to those individuals who have progressively lost GJH due to increasing age.

The questionnaire consists of five items:

(Q1)   *'Can you now (or could you ever) place your hands flat on the floor without bending your knees?' (Yes/No);*

(Q2)   *'Can you now (or could you ever) bend your thumb to touch your forearm?' (Yes/No);*

(Q3)   *'As a child did you amuse your friends by contorting your body into strange shapes or could you do the splits* (Figs. 3.2 and 3.3)*?' (Yes/No);*

(Q4)   *'As a child or teenager did your shoulder or kneecap dislocate on more than one occasion?' (Yes/No);*

(Q5)   *'Do you consider yourself to be double-jointed?' (Yes/No).*

In 2005, Lamari et al. analysed the range of articular movements of 1120 children of both sexes between

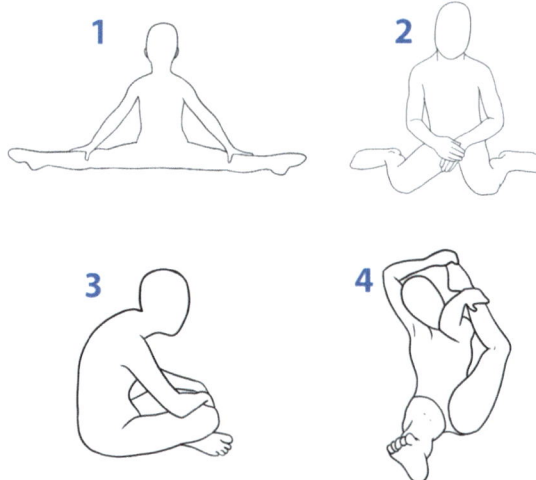

Fig. 3.2 Ilustration of atypical and characteristic positions of individuals with JH when sitting (Mateus Lamari's doctoral thesis, 2021)

the ages of 4 and 7 (Lamari et al. 2005). These children exhibited significant changes in body composition in this age range. The authors suggested that this process probably reflected the redistribution of subcutaneous body fat and muscle tissue. Boys have greater body density than girls, and, consequently, have a lower percentage of body fat (Malina and Bouchard 1991). These observations also justify the conclusion of previous studies that females have greater joint mobility then males at any specific age (Lamari and Lamari 2016; Malina et al. 2021).

In their extensive investigation in 2005, Lamari et al. (2005) found that mobility decreased with increasing age, among the 1120 children, even in the narrow range of their ages. On the basis of these observations, it was possible to confirm that the parameters and criteria used to assess joint mobility were applicable to all age groups,

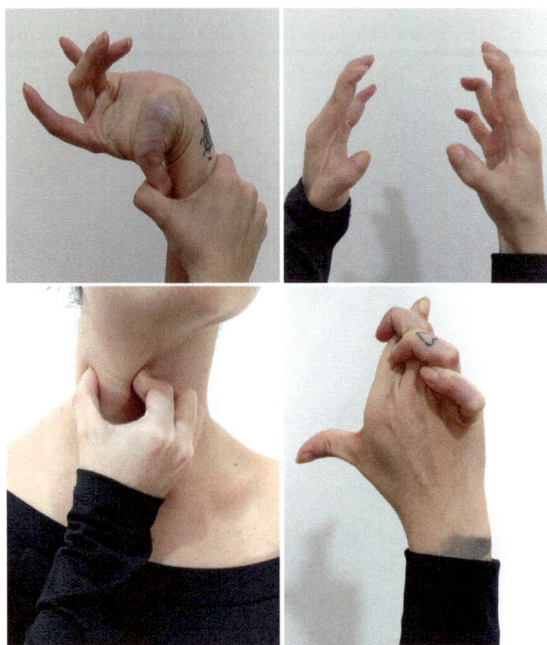

Fig. 3.3 Body contortions into strange shapes

including adults and children. In this context, Lamari et al. (2005) also suggested that it would be appropriate for the current scoring scales to be revised.

Adjustments to the Beighton score have been proposed based on age group and anatomical location of the characteristic under evaluation. Malfait et al. (2017) suggested changes to the Beighton scoring method based on the periods of life, with a positive score of 6 for children and prepubescent adolescents, a score of 5 for pubescent individuals and up to 50 years of age and a score of 4 for those aged 50 years or older. Castori et al. (2017) published criteria for the identification of JH based on the location of the affected region, in five or more anatomical regions (the four limbs and the axial skeleton). Peripheral joint hypermobility (PJH) is a potentially mild form identified only in the hands and/or feet. Localised joint hypermobilty (LJH) is recorded when only one joint (large or small, unilaterally or bilaterally) is affected. LJH may be inherited or acquired due to trauma, joint disease, surgery or exercise training.

It is noteworthy that, throughout the history regarding the method of identification of the characteristics of GJH, the majority of modifications have been made since 1973. Nevertheless, an alternative method of quantication of mobility has not yet been proposed. For this reason, the scoring system established by Beighton et al. (1973) remains the most frequently used in the current literature. Although adjustments were proposed in 2017, the methodology of the original score was preserved (Beighton and Horan 1970).

References

Beighton PH, Horan FT. Dominant inheritance in familial generalised articular hypermobility. J Bone Joint Surg Br. 1970;52:145–7.

Beighton P, Solomon I, Soskolne L. Articular mobility in an African population. Ann Rheum Dis. 1973;32:413–8.

Carter C, Wilkinson LE. Persistent joint laxity and congenital dislocation of the hypermobility. J Bone Joint Surg Br. 1964;46B:40–5.

Castori M, Tinkle B, Levy H, Grahame R, Malfait F, Hakim A. A framework for the classification of joint hypermobility and related conditions. Am J Med Genet C Semin Med Genet. 2017;175:148–57.

Hakim AJ, Grahame R. A simple questionnaire to detect hypermobility: an adjunct to the assessment of patients with diffuse musculoskeletal pain. Int J Clin Pract. 2003;57:163–6.

Lamari NM, Lamari MM. Characterization of Brazilian children with joint hypermobility. Int J Physiatry. 2016;2:011.

Lamari NM, Chueire AG, Cordeiro JA. Analysis of joint mobility patterns among preschool children. São Paulo Med J. 2005;123:119–23.

Malina RM, Bouchard C. Growth, maturation, and physical activity. Champaign: Human Kinetics; 1991. Chap. 2. p. 11–20.

Malina RM, Martinho DV, Santos JV, Silva MJC, Kozieł SM. Growth and maturity status of female soccer players: a narrative review. Int J Environ Res Public Health. 2021;18:1448.

Malfait F, Francomano C, Byers P, Belmont J, Berglund B, Black J, et al. The 2017 international classification of the Ehlers-Danlos syndromes. Am J Med Genet C Semin Med Genet. 2017;175:8–26.

4

The Heterogeneity of Joint Hypermobility

Classification and Nomenclature of Symptomatic Hypermobility

In the last decade, growing attention has been given to joint hypermobility (JH) and related disorders. The new nosology for Ehlers-Danlos syndromes (EDS), which is the best known and probably the most common genetic disorder involving JH, identifies more than 20 different causative genes. It is stressed that there is a need for a single set of criteria to replace previous criteria, specifically for EDS hypermobility type (EDS-HT) and JH syndrome (JHS). These conditions were considered the two most overlapping conditions in the current nosology for EDS and a new entity has been proposed, designated the hypermobile Ehlers-Danlos syndrome (hEDS) (Castori et al. 2017).

© The Author(s), under exclusive license to Springer Nature Switzerland AG 2023
N. Lamari and P. Beighton, *Hypermobility in Medical Practice*, In Clinical Practice, https://doi.org/10.1007/978-3-031-34914-0_4

The concept of a spectrum of pathogenic manifestations related to JH was also concerning the categories of pleiotropic syndromes with JH. Thus, for several disorders in the hypermobility spectrum diagnostic labels were proposed for patients with symptomatic JH that do not correspond to any other syndromes involving JH (Castori et al. 2017). Individuals with JH could then be classified as asymptomatic or having a well-defined syndrome involving JH, including hypermobile EDS. Similarly, hypermobility spectrum disorders (HSD) are comprised of individuals with symptomatic JH that do not meet the criteria/diagnosis for a specific syndrome. These HSDs are a group of clinical conditions related to JH that are distinguishable from hEDS and other syndromes involving JH, since the phenotypes of HSDs are generally limited to the musculoskeletal system.

Involvement of the musculoskeletal system is considered in the presence of one or more manifestations secondary to JH, such as trauma, pain, degenerative joint and bone disease, or manifestations of neurological or orthopedic development. In this way, there are some individuals with asymptomatic JH, in addition to those who are symptomatic and have HSD (Castori et al. 2017).

The proposed new nosology for EDS (Malfait et al. 2017) and the structure for the classification of hypermobility and related conditions (Castori et al. 2017) represent notable scientific contributions but these still pose difficulties for clinicians. These problems are beyond the difficulties inherent in the vast number of preclinical and clinical manifestations, which vary considerably among affected individuals. Moreover, there is greater difficulty in the analysis of syndromic manifestations in children and preadolescents.

Joint Hypermobility Syndrome Terminology

Children and pre-adolescents with musculoskeletal pain, without other signs and symptoms and JH are often seen in clinical practice by pediatricians and other healthcare professionals. It is relevant that, in these age groups, the manifestations related to JH are far short of the diagnosis of exclusion for hEDS. according to the proposal by Castori et al. (2017) Frequently, the only associated manifestation is severe pain in the legs that begins in childhood or preadolescence, with many disabling episodes that leave the patient, parents, and pediatrician with a sensation of being powerless.

In this situation, it is relevant for pediatricians, dentists, physical educators, and physiotherapists to correlate the manifestation of "growing pains" (Sperotto et al. 2014; Shim 2015) with the characteristic of JH. It is also important to identify the condition early, as a significant percentage of adults with JH report a history of "growing pains" and disabilities. Thereafter they may become adults with chronic, disabling pain (Lamari et al. 2020). It is relevant however that many children with growing pains do not have JH.

This symptom of "growing pains" poses considerable difficulty for parents, as it can occur in the form of periodic episodes over the years, affect the child for hours or a few days, and disappear for no apparent reason. However, these same children may present with other undervalued or misunderstood manifestations, such as difficulty during recreational activities at or outside of school and difficulty in writing due to the positioning of the pencil between the thumb and index finger (Bravo 2010; Artigues-Cano and Bird 2014) For these reasons, the modification of JHS terminology has hindered the understanding of manifestations in this age group.

Ross and Grahame (2011) stated that there is no consensus among researchers regarding differences in the nomenclatures as to whether JH is only a less severe type of EDS III, which according to Castori et al. (2017) is currently termed "HSD". This concern has culminated in the important denomination of HSDs for individuals with manifestations that resemble those of hEDS but who do not meet the diagnostic criteria. However, there are no diagnostic criteria for the condition in children and preadolescents with symptomatic hypermobility, the frequency of which is high in the general population (Clinch et al. 2011; Sohrbeck-Nøhr et al. 2014; Lamari et al. 2020).

Joint Hypermobility Syndrome Diagnostic Criteria

The exclusion of the JHS terminology has made the early diagnosis of JH in symptomatic children and preadolescents unviable, leaving a gap for those individuals who do not meet the diagnostic criteria for HSDs or asymptomatic JH. Moreover, the complexity of the analysis of the diagnostic criteria for hEDS by clinicians has led to the continual underdiagnosis of hEDS and HSDs, especially in children and adolescents. In this way, many affected persons miss out on the opportunity for preventive care for other problems that could emerge and require the promotion of physical health, as the joints may become compromised due to inadequate body mechanics.

The medical profession is now seeing adults with insurmountable disabling pain that began in childhood and was overlooked. Such individuals become adults with degenerative joint processes and deformities, such as flat feet, valgus foot, scoliosis, the reactivation or accentuation of physiological curves of the spinal column, genu recurvatum and rotation of the femoral heads (Marino et al. 2004; Adib et al. 2005; Berglund et al. 2005; Groh and Herrera 2009; Shirley et al. 2012; Tobias et al. 2013; Czaprowski 2014; Daniels et al. 2016; Ericson and Wolman 2017). In particular, disabling pain (Coster et al. 2005; Groh and Herrera 2009; Castori et al. 2010; Chopra et al. 2017; Tinkle et al. 2017) may affect daily, instrumental, recreational, sports, and occupational activities (Schmidt et al. 2017; Nathan et al. 2018; Gyer et al. 2018) This situation could have been avoided or attenuated when the signs and symptoms were less evident and not suggestive of a disorder. In this situation this condition, the denomination "Joint Hypermobility Syndrome" may be used in children and preadolescents with JH, after the exclusion of other collagen conditions.

It is important that pediatricians, dentists, physical educators, and physiotherapists understand in a timely manner the problems that these children and preadolescents might have, what the implications are, and when and how to refer them for multidisciplinary care due to the possible changes in body mechanics in childhood (Engelbert et al. 2003; Tobias et al. 2013; Czaprowski 2014; Daniels et al. 2016) Special care may be needed until the end of the adolescent growth spurt (Carrascosa et al. 2018). Moreover, guidance regarding care during recreational and sports activities is also necessary because of these frailties.

When there is awareness of the implications of the instabilities in body mechanics, the patient may be able to recognize his/her limits with regards to strength and endurance. This approach would change the lifestyle and course of the condition in these patients, who require medical management, since they were born with hypermobile joints. JH is in their genes and linked to the production of abnormal collagen or a similar protein. This deficiency makes the tissues of the body less robust and, therefore, less capable of coping with the physical tensions of daily living (Ross and Grahame 2011).

Hypermobile joints can progress to early degenerative processes in the cartilage which is essential to smooth movements between adjacent bones. Such wear precedes the onset of painful osteoarthritis, can emerge in young adults (Gürer et al. 2018; Saltzman et al. 2018; Lamari et al. 2020).

Affected children cannot be analyzed on a basis of syndromic factors which are predominantly found in adults. Consequently, hypermobility and pain in children may be denominated as "growing pains" and leave affected children to suffer due to the lack the correct diagnosis. Equally, problems may arise concerning the proper management which involves prevention and health promotion measures (El-Metwally et al. 2006; Viswanathan and Khubchandani 2008; Peterson et al. 2018).

Specific Diagnostic Criteria for Infants, Children, and Preadolescents

Affected children exhibit disabling episodes of pain in the legs over the years. These evolve into chronic pain that might make them unable to participate in scholastic, recreational, and sports activities. These problems may also persist during academic and occupational activities throughout the lifecycle.

Many families look for the diagnosis and treatment of JH in their children. With the advent of the internet, parents currently have access to information that describes the situation of their children. In this way, they can obtain some relief and/or assistance from the few healthcare providers who are prepared to offer appropriate management of these children, especially until the adolescent growth spurt.

In these children, especially infants, the diagnosis could be made through an inspection and physical examination involving palpation and passive mobilization of the joints, with a maximum duration of two minutes. In older children, the use of the Beighton score (Beighton et al. 1973) with a physical examination of the hips, shoulders, and feet is relevant. Moreover, there is considerable importance in the "handshake sign", recognized by the limpness of the hand, which differs from that of other children (Lamari et al. 2020) and is frequently reported by parents.

Other components of the natural history of adults with JH are the occurrence of benign delayed neuropsychomotor development (Davidovitch et al. 1994; Ghibellini et al. 2015; Radmilović et al. 2016) and an inexplicable difficulty breastfeeding (Chaplin et al. 2016; Wood et al. 2016), supposedly due to the weakness of orofacial muscles (Pires et al. 2012; D'Onofrio 2019), A high-arched palate (Bradburn and Hall 1995; Marsili et al. 2020), a long and/or flaccid tongue (Surendran et al. 2012), hypermobile larynx and trachea (Cesare et al. 2019), and a mouth-breathing pattern (Melo et al. 2015; Azevedo et al. 2018) are other manifestations that can lead to a diagnosis of JH.

It is important for pediatricians, dentists, physical educators, and physiotherapists in both public and private services to have knowledge regarding the minimal criteria for the identification of JH. With this information, healthcare providers could offer support and clarification to parents and family members. There is also a need for qualified healthcare professionals to provide specialized care for these patients. This would naturally lead to a change in the culture of different fields of health, enabling affected individuals to become hypermobile adults without drastic orthopedic problems, such as fallen arches, deviation of the vertebral axis and alignment of the knees. These also include a gait pattern with hip rotation (Marino et al. 2004; Adib et al. 2005; Groh and Herrera 2009; Scheper et al. 2016; Ericson and Wolman 2017) and consequent degenerative joints with osteoarthritis that can emerge silently even in young people.

Most people with JH and associated manifestations, excluding other disorders of collagen or a similar protein, would benefit from the early intervention of pediatricians, dentists, physical educators, and physiotherapists. Health promotion and the prevention of changes in body mechanics that affect the face, spinal column, and upper and lower limbs are relevant. Thus, the establishment of minimal diagnostic criteria in routine clinical and kinesiofunctional evaluations beginning in childhood is important. This approach could change the future of affected individuals who have a wide range of tissue frailties, from the oral cavity to the feet.

References

Adib N, Davies K, Grahame R, Woo P, Murray KJ. Joint hypermobility syndrome in childhood. A not so benign multisystem disorder? Rheumatology (Oxford). 2005;44:744–50.

Artigues-Cano I, Bird HA. Hypermobility and proprioception in the finger joints of flautists. J Clin Rheumatol. 2014;20:203–8.

Azevedo ND, Lima JC, Furlan RMMM, Motta AR. Tongue pressure measurement in children with mouth-breathing behaviour. J Oral Rehabil. 2018;45:612–7.

Beighton P, Solomon I, Soskolne L. Articular mobility in an African population. Ann Rheum Dis. 1973;32:413–8.

Berglund B, Nordström G, Hagberg C, Mattiasson AC. Foot pain and disability in individuals with Ehlers-Danlos syndrome (EDS): impact on daily life activities. Disabil Rehabil. 2005;27:164–9.

Bradburn JM, Hall BD. Spondyloepimetaphyseal dysplasia with joint laxity (SEMDJL): clinical and radiological findings in a Guatemalan patient. Am J Med Genet. 1995;59:234–7.

Bravo JF. Síndrome de Ehlers-Danlos tipo III, llamado también Síndrome de Hiperlaxitud Articular (SHA): Epidemiología y manifestaciones clínicas. Rev Chil Reumatol. 2010;26:194–202.

Carrascosa A, Yeste D, Moreno-Galdó A, Gussinyé M, Ferrández A, Clemente M et al. Pubertal growth of 1453 healthy children according to age at pubertal growth spurt onset. The Barcelona longitudinal growth study. An Pediatr (Barc). 2018;89:144–52.

Castori M, Camerota F, Celletti C, Danese C, Santilli V, Saraceni VM, et al. Natural history and manifestations of the hypermobility type Ehlers-Danlos syndrome: a pilot study on 21 patients. Am J Med Genet A. 2010;152A:556–64.

Castori M, Tinkle B, Levy H, Grahame R, Malfait F, Hakim A. A framework for the classification of joint hypermobility and related conditions. Am J Med Genet C Semin Med Genet. 2017;175:148–57.

Cesare AE, Rafer LC, Myler CS, Brennan KB. Anesthetic management for Ehlers-Danlos syndrome, hypermobility type complicated by local anesthetic allergy: a case report. Am J Case Rep. 2019;20:39–42.

Chaplin J, Kelly J, Kildea S. Maternal perceptions of breastfeeding difficulty after caesarean section with regional anaesthesia: a qualitative study. Women Birth. 2016;29:144–52.

Chopra P, Tinkle P, Hamonet C, Brock I, Gompel A, Bulbena A, et al. Pain Management in the Ehlers-Danlos syndromes. Am J Med Genet C Semin Med Genet. 2017;175:212–9.

Clinch J, Deere K, Sayers A, Palmer S, Riddoch C, Tobias JH, et al. Epidemiology of generalized joint laxity (hypermobility) in fourteen-year-old children from the UK: a population-based evaluation. Arthritis Rheum. 2011;63:2819–27.

Czaprowski D. Generalised joint hypermobility in caucasian girls with idiopathic scoliosis: relation with age, curve size, and curve pattern. Scientific World J. 2014;2014:1–6.

Daniels AH, DePasse JM, Kamal RN. Orthopaedic surgeon burnout: Diagnosis, treatment, and prevention. J Am Acad Orthop Surg. 2016;24:213–9.

Davidovitch M, Tirosh E, Tal Y. The relationship between joint hypermobility and neurodevelopmental attributes in elementary school children. J Child Neurol. 1994;9:417–9.

De Coster PJ, Van den Berghe LI, Martens LC. Generalized joint hypermobility and temporomandibular disorders: inherited connective tissue disease as a model with maximum expression. J Orofac Pain. 2005;19:47–57.

D'Onofrio L. Oral dysfunction as a cause of malocclusion. Orthod Craniofac Res. 2019;22(Suppl 1):43–8.

El-Metwally A, Salminen JJ, Auvinen A, Kautiainen H, Mikkelsson M. Risk factors for traumatic and non-traumatic lower limb pain among preadolescents: a population-based study of Finnish schoolchildren. BMC Musculoskelet Disord. 2006;7:3.

Engelbert RH, Bank RA, Sakkers RJ, Helders PJ, Beemer FA, Uiterwaal CS. Pediatric generalized joint hypermobility with and without musculoskeletal complaints: a localized or systemic disorder? Pediatrics. 2003;111:e248–54.

Ericson WB Jr, Wolman R. Orthopaedic management of the Ehlers-Danlos syndromes. Am J Med Genet C Semin Med Genet. 2017;175:188–94.

Ghibellini G, Brancati F, Castori M. Neurodevelopmental attributes of joint hypermobility syndrome/Ehlers-Danlos syndrome, hypermobility type: update and perspectives. Am J Med Genet C Semin Med Genet. 2015;169C:107–16.

Groh MM, Herrera J. A comprehensive review of hip labral tears. Curr Ver Musculoskelet Med. 2009;2:105–7.

Gürer G, Bozbas GT, Tuncer T, Unubol AI, Ucar UG, Memetoglu OI. Frequency of joint hypermobility in Turkish patients with knee osteoarthritis: a cross sectional multicenter study. Int J Rheum Dis. 2018;21:1787–92.

Gyer G, Michael J, Inklebarger J. Occupational hand injuries: a current review of the prevalence and proposed prevention strategies for physical therapists and similar healthcare professionals. J Integr Med. 2018;16:84–9.

Lamari MM, Lamari NM, Medeiros MP, Pavarino EC. Signos y Síntomas en niños y adolescentes con Hipermovilidad Articular: Un estudio transversal cuantitativo observacional. Rev Chil Reumatol. 2020;36:42–53.

Malfait F, Francomano C, Byers P, Belmont J, Berglund B, Black J, et al. The 2017 international classification of the Ehlers-Danlos syndromes. Am J Med Genet Part C Semin Med Genet. 2017;175:8–26.

Marino LHC, Lamari N, Marino NW Jr. HA nos joelhos da criança. Arq Ciênc Saúde. 2004;11:124–7.

Marsili L, Overwater E, Hanna N, et al. Phenotypic spectrum of TGFB3 disease-causing variants in a Dutch-French cohort and first report of a homozygous patient. Clin Genet. 2020;97:723–30.

Melo AC, Gomes Ade O, Cavalcanti AS, Silva HJ. Acoustic rhinometry in mouth breathing patients: a systematic review. Braz J Otorhinolaryngol. 2015;81:212–8. https://doi.org/10.1016/j.bjorl.2014.12.007.

Nathan JA, Davies K, Swaine I. Hypermobility and sports injury. BMJ Open Sport Exerc Med. 2018;4:e000366.

Peterson B, Coda A, Pacey V, Hawke F. Physical and mechanical therapies for lower limb symptoms in children with hypermobility spectrum disorder and hypermobile Ehlers-Danlos syndrome: a systematic review. J Foot Ankle Res. 2018;11:59.

Pires SC, Giugliani ER, Caramez da Silva F. Influence of the duration of breastfeeding on quality of muscle function during mastication in preschoolers: a cohort study. BMC Public Health. 2012;12:934.

Radmilović G, Matijević V, Zavoreo I. Comparison of psychomotor development screening test and clinical assessment of psychomotor development. Acta Clin Croat. 2016;55:600–6.

Ross J, Grahame R. Joint hypermobility syndrome. BMJ. 2011;342: c7167.

Saltzman BM, Leroux TS, Verma NN, Romeo AA. Glenohumeral osteoarthritis in the young patient. J Am Acad Orthop Surg. 2018;26:e361–70.

Scheper MC, Juul-Kristensen B, Rombaut L, Rameckers EA, Verbunt J, Engelbert RH. Disability in adolescents and adults diagnosed with hypermobility-related disorders: a meta-analysis. Arch Phys Med Rehabil. 2016;97:2174–87.

Schmidt H, Pedersen TL, Junge T, Engelbert R, Juul-Kristensen B. Hypermobility in adolescent athletes: pain, functional ability, quality of life, and musculoskeletal injuries. J Orthop Sports Phys Ther. 2017;47:792–800.

Shim KS. Pubertal growth and epiphyseal fusion. Ann Pediatr Endocrinol Metab. 2015;20:8–12.

Shirley ED, Demaio M, Bodurtha J. Ehlers-danlos syndrome in orthopaedics: etiology, diagnosis, and treatment implications. Sports Health. 2012;4:394–403.

Sohrbeck-Nøhr O, Kristensen JH, Boyle E, Remvig L, Juul-Kristensen B. Generalized joint hypermobility in childhood is a possible risk for the development of joint pain in adolescence: a cohort study. BMC Pediatr. 2014;14:302.

Sperotto F, Balzarin M, Parolin M, Monteforte N, Vittadello F, Zulian F. Joint hypermobility, growing pain and obesity are mutually exclusive as causes of musculoskeletal pain in schoolchildren. Clin Exp Rheumatol. 2014;32:131–6.

Surendran S, Thomas E, Asokan S. Hypermobile tongue. Br Dent J. 2012;212:55–6.

Tinkle B, Castori M, Berglund B, Cohen H, Grahame R, Kazkaz H, et al. Hypermobile Ehlers–Danlos syndrome (a.k.a. Ehlers–Danlos Syndrome Type III and Ehlers–Danlos syndrome hypermobility type): clinical description and natural history. Am J Med Genet C Semin Med Genet. 2017;175:48–69.

Tobias JH, Deere K, Palmer S, Clark EM, Clinch J. Joint hypermobility is a risk factor for musculoskeletal pain during adolescence: findings of a prospective cohort study. Arthritis Rheum. 2013;65:1107–15.

Viswanathan V, Khubchandani RP. Joint hypermobility and growing pains in school children. Clin Exp Rheumatol. 2008;26:962–6.

Wood NK, Woods NF, Blackburn ST, Sanders EA. Interventions that enhance breastfeeding initiation, duration, and exclusivity: a systematic review. MCN Am J Matern Child Nurs. 2016;41:299–307.

5

Biomechanical Aspects of Joint Hypermobility

Negative Factors in Joint Biomechanics

Joint hypermobility alters the biomechanics of the loco-motor system due to ligament failure, a lack of adequate tension for the promotion of stability. There is decreased strength, fatigue and muscle weakness. These manifestations interfere with the stability of the vertebral bodies, both statically and dynamically. The range of motion in any joint depends on a variety of factors, including muscle tone, elasticity of ligaments and joint capsules, and the shape of bone contours (Beighton et al. 2012).

The main determinants of joint laxity were identified in the studies by Johns and Wright (1962), who greatly contributed to the understanding of body structure effectiveness in joint mechanics. These authors used an arthrographic technique to determine the proportional contribution of each tissue layer to joint stiffness. They observed that nonlinear elasticity and plasticity accounted

© The Author(s), under exclusive license to Springer Nature
Switzerland AG 2023
N. Lamari and P. Beighton, *Hypermobility in Medical Practice*,
In Clinical Practice, https://doi.org/10.1007/978-3-031-34914-0_5

for most stiffness, with the elasticity being twice as important as plasticity. It is relevant that muscles play a significant role in supporting skeletal structures (Kendal et al. 2007). The medical implications of joint laxity have been reviewed by Beighton, Grahame and Bird in successive editions of their monograph "Hypermobility of Joints" (Beighton et al. 2012).

The contributions of Bird (1983) to epidemiological and clinical issues highlight the relevance of the structures that determine joint mobility, such as the shape of the articular bone surfaces, collagen organization, joint capsules, neuromuscular tone, along with overlying tissues and their degree of stretching. In addition, a tensile force is exerted by the muscles and tendons in almost all positions of the joints. Joints are more mobile in their intermediate proximity than at their extremity (Bird 1983).

Bones provide mechanical support through a framework consisting of a collagen matrix on which calcium salts are deposited and this is responsible for their strength. The tendon is a fibrous structure that transmits muscle strength and generates movement, while ligaments are the bundles of resistant fibers, which are fundamental in controlling movement by promoting stability to the joint (Enoka 2000).

Stability of a ligament is obtained by the strength and elasticity of the collagen, which varies between individuals according to the inherited collagen structure (Bird and Knight 2012). According to Dutton (2012), collagen plays an important role in maintaining the structural integrity of various tissues and is responsible for the resistance to tension, firmness, and connective tissue in support of the body. In hypermobility, collagen alteration directly affects the ligaments, allowing the joints to advance beyond the degree of movement, which is usually regarded as being normal.

The human body adapts to many different situations. It sustains itself by tensing the muscles in search of balance and support with hypermobile structures, as a way to compensate for the hypermobility of joints. The evolution of body movements, with their specific functions, occurs as a consequence of adaptive mechanical responses from the musculoskeletal system tissues. It is a natural interaction of form and function and can be defined as a modification of an organism or its parts, which makes it more suitable for existing in its environmental conditions (Pinheiro et al. 2013). In this way, bones are also subjected to the adaptive characteristics of loads and forces that are imposed upon them throughout skeletal development.

Adaptation of skeletal muscles occurs by passive and active adjustments of forces for the effective muscle activities of contraction and relaxation. The combination of these mechanical properties and the behaviour of musculoskeletal tissues is relevant to the understanding of the mechanical functioning of joint mobility (Kłodowski and Rantalainen 2015). In this context, biomechanical studies indicate that all human body movements are a result of the orchestration of forces around joints (Purvis 2017) and that the architectural body frame displays a physiological response to these forces (Levangie and Norkin 2011). Just as anatomy is influenced by mechanical force, gravitational force also influences musculoskeletal architecture. Skeleton development is influenced by the activity of these forces during the developmental processes at different stages of life. Approximately 10% of the human skeleton is remodelled every year and remodelled every 10 years by stress patterns to which it is exposed (Bradley and O'Donnell 2007).

Constant irritative pressures, such as postural deformities, cause bone atrophy, while the intermittent stresses of normal activities can favour bone growth, such as walking, sitting, and lifting. Thus, appropriate weight bearing stimulates osteogenesis, which is influenced by the piezoelectric effect (Whiting and Zernicke 2008).

Among the various intervening factors in joint mechanics are the genetic, biological, hormonal, and nutritional aspects, along with stress. In this context it is relevant that bone growth outside a living organism adapts to the artificial forces which are present in the tissue culture (Purvis 2017).

Joint Stability and Instability

A lesion in any component of the musculoskeletal system can modify the mechanical interactions and can cause degradation, instability, or incapacity for movement. Conversely, the alteration, manipulation, and adequate control of the mechanical environment can contribute to the prevention of injuries, correction of abnormalities, and the acceleration of healing and rehabilitation (Lu and Chang 2012).

Joint instability is frequent among hypermobile individuals and can compromise movements with a greater risk of injuries and consequent dysfunction (Steinmann et al. 2003; Ericson and Wolman 2017). Joint stability is the capacity to maintain or control the position or movement of a joint. It depends upon coordinated actions of the surrounding tissues for static stability and on the neuromuscular system for dynamic stability. Joint stability is influenced by muscle strength, muscle insertion angle, length-tension relationships, and force–velocity. Static joint stability is provided by the joint capsules, ligaments, and bony parts that articulate (Nordin and Frankel 2012). The requirements are for body support, which minimize muscular compensation and protect the joints, ligaments and tendons (Abrantes 2006).

Joint instability occurs when tissues such as muscles, ligaments, and capsules lose their physiological properties, as occurs in hypermobile individuals. Therefore, mobility does not meet the normal standards, as there is a tendency to degenerative processes due to irregular joint movement. In this way joint stability is the ability to control the mobility that provides security (Fig. 5.1) (Abrantes 2006).

Flexibility in Joint Hypermobility

Joint mobility is directly dependent on the structures by which it is constituted and surrounded (Rodrigues 1998). The motion of a joint depends on the shape of contact surfaces and passive stabilization and flexibility

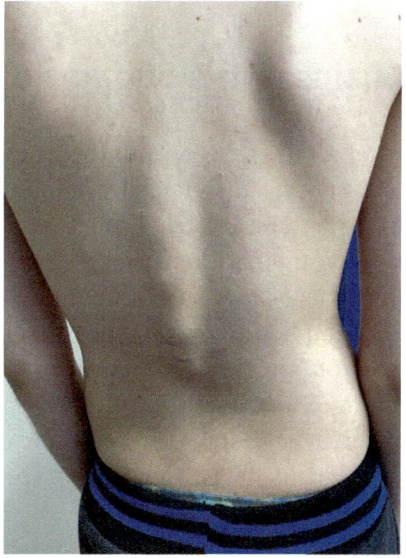

Fig. 5.1 Degenerative processes in the spine due to irregular joint movement while sitting

of ligaments. Joint flexibility requires elasticity of skeletal muscles and connective tissues depending on the joint type. Spherical joints, such as hip and shoulder joints, allow for a greater range of motion, while hinge joints limit motion along only one axis.

To some extent, joint flexibility is determined by age, gender, and body temperature (Purvis 2017). Limited flexibility is frequently associated with a greater incidence of muscle injuries. However, hypermobility increases joint instability, which is characterized by flexibility and increases the risk of various injuries (Kassel 2018). Active flexibility is dependent on muscle strength which improves flexibility and influences physical performance (Malina and Bouchard 1991; Malina et al. 2021). Mechanical properties of collagenous tissues, which surround the skeletal system, are passive structures that do not produce active movement (Purvis 2017).

Muscle Chains in the Support of Joints

The support of body weight and the consequent segmental stabilization are maintained dynamically by muscular actions and statically by ligaments. These factors are important for the maintenance of the physiological segmental position, preventing functional alterations. Ligament laxity implies a low afferent regulation to muscle stretch receptors and reduces proprioception. For these reasons, joint movements are impaired in persons with generalized joint hypermobility since motor coordination and stability fundamentally depend on proprioceptive feedback (Chiodelli et al. 2015).

Muscle chains are a set of muscles that are in the same region and with similar orientation. They are usually polyarticular, behaving like one muscle and overlap each other. Thus, every attempt at local correction will generate compensation at a distance. The tension of a muscle chain results in a tendency for internal rotation of the limbs. In these chains, the muscles form a passage for the lines of force that run through the body. There are chains of static and dynamic muscles; the latter are used for main movements, where the amount of connective tissue is smaller and the muscle tone is lower. Thus, muscles can become extremely flaccid and hypotonic, especially in the abdominal musculature (Mézières 1984).

In this context, when one member of a muscle chain is affected, all the other muscles of the same chain are similarly involved. The muscle-ligament hyperelasticity causes a series of reactions that leads to segmental instability. In this situation, the hyperelastic muscles of hypermobile individuals alter the segmental positioning due to the lack of dynamic and static control normally generated by the action of these muscles and ligaments, which no longer have a stabilizing function.

Support and Stabilization of the Spine

The vertebral column, regarded as a cantilever beam that supports stable and mobile loads, has the functions of support, movement, flexibility, and maintenance of balance for the body. The primary function of the spine is to provide the body with longitudinal rigidity, allowing movement between its parts. The spine also constitutes a firm base for supporting contiguous anatomical structures, such as ribs and abdominal muscles, thereby contributing to the maintenance of the body cavities. The intervertebral discs separate the vertebral bodies, allowing the vertebrae to bend over each other. One of the most relevant aspects of the intervertebral disc biomechanics is the pressure variation that occurs in its structure in various postures. Flexion is the most pronounced movement of the spine (Whiting and Zernicke 2008). Individuals with hypermobility in this region usually experience radicular pain due to disc failure at L4–L5 or piriformis syndrome (irritation of the sciatic nerve by the piriformis muscle in the buttocks) or both (Ericson and Wolman 2017).

The cervical spine is the most mobile region of the entire spine and has the most elaborate and specialized muscular system. It supports and moves the head and protects the neural and vascular structures. It is estimated that it moves about 600 times per hour, or every six seconds. Cervical spinal structures are responsible for absorbing impacts and dispersing mechanical energy and they are important in the initiation of degenerative processes in this region (Kapandji 2000).

Flexion of the cervical spine is limited by the posterior longitudinal ligament, vertebral elements, and limited elasticity of the fascia of the extensor muscles. Excessive extension of the spine is limited by direct contact of the vertebral laminae, interfacet joints, and the posterosuperior spinous processes. Support of the cervical spine is maintained by the action of the posterior muscles, mainly the trapezius muscle and deep musculature that connects one vertebral body to another (Amadio et al. 1999).

Superior fibers of the trapezius and levator scapulae muscle are partly responsible for some movements of the cervical spine and scapula. These muscles can easily be overloaded by weakness and underuse of the other cervical and scapular stabilizing muscles. In the absence of this division of labour, the tension of these muscles increases and trigger points (nodules) occur, causing and/or aggravating pain in pre-existing degenerative processes (Kapandji 2000).

Cervical muscle weaknesses and distended, loose, or overstretched muscles in a hypermobile individual prevent the correct alignment of the cervical spine, leading to the anterior or lateral displacement of the head. A relatively anterior position of the head in relation to the shoulders can overload the posterior structures of the cervical spine. For such individuals, an ideal posture would be for their ears to be aligned with their shoulders. In this way, the head would be 1/3rd posterior and 2/3rd anterior in relation to the shoulder line. When sitting in front of a computer or a book, with the head in front, the entire head weight is in front of the shoulder line, generating overload on the muscles, ligaments, joints, and intervertebral discs in the posterior cervical region (Chiodelli et al. 2015).

Due to the high flexibility of the cervical spine, forward flexion of the head is possible. These movements are a function of mobility in rotational movements, extending backward, or because of the activity of spinal joints, which also help protect the spinal cord. The intervertebral disc assists in mobility and acts as a "shock absorber" for the vertebrae. Over the years, the disc can be compromised by varying degrees of degeneration, becoming thinner or even shifting from its natural position between the vertebrae. The result of this phenomenon can be cervical spine pain (Mckhael et al. 2020). Individuals with joint hypermobility may present craniocervical instability, an Arnold-Chiari malformation, or cervical spondylosis (Ericson and Wolman 2017).

Support and Stabilization of the Pelvis and Hips

A total of 22 muscles act on the hip joint, and there is a high degree of mobility with stability provided to the joint by its architecture and ligamentous support. Control and positioning of the pelvis and hip, considering the transversal or horizontal balance of the pelvis, is maintained by forces that act on the pelvis, such as the downward force of body weight and the upward reaction force from the ground. Combined muscular actions of the anterior musculature of the trunk synchronized with the posterior musculature of the limbs also acts in its stabilization. Additionally, efficient function is determined by the posterior musculature of the trunk synchronized with the anterior musculature of the limbs and by concomitant actions of the lateral pelvic muscles. Transverse stability requires the pelvic muscle actions to be free of shortening, weakness, or any other factor that limits movement (Kapandji 2000). Hip pain is common in the Elhers-Danlos Syndrome (EDS) and can occur because of sacroiliac subluxation of the iliotibial band over the greater trochanter, which can lead to trochanteric bursitis due to joint instability (Ericson and Wolman 2017).

Support and Stabilization of the Knee

The knee is the largest and most mechanically stressed joint of the human body. Since it is subjected to a high mechanical stress during its support function, many injuries are associated with it, including total and partial ligament ruptures, bone fractures, osteochondral lesions, fissures and damage in the menisci, among others. The biomechanical functionality of the knee joint originates from a complex interaction between its structural components. Thus, any damage to these components can lead to imbalance in the natural biomechanics of the knee and promote deterioration of the entire joint system.

Marino et al. (2004) reported that 12.5% of children have hyperextensible knees, and that children with generalized hypermobility (GJH) have joint pain as a primary complaint (Fatoye et al. 2009). Knee injuries are common in individuals with joint hypermobility (Kerr et al. 2000) and in soccer players (Myer et al. 2008), anterior cruciate ligament injury predominates (Ramesh et al. 2005).

Support and Stabilization of the Ankle and Foot

The ankle joint is decisive in the transmission of force from and to the body during weight bearing and other tasks. The magnitude of these forces can be up to 10 times the body weight during some types of running. Even small structural misalignments or injuries can lead to chronic and intense orthopaedic problems (Norkin and White 2017). Mechanical considerations of the ankle and foot injuries explain their frequency and ankle joint injuries are the most common injury in some sports. Extreme motion in either direction can be injurious but is less frequent than injury caused by laterally directed forces that result in inversion or eversion. Inversion injuries account for 85% of all ankle injuries (Whiting and Zernicke 2008).

Musculoskeletal injuries by excessive motion and inadequate muscle control are often attributed to a flatfoot (Fig. 5.2). However, many of the speculated differences in mechanics and control between normal and flat feet have not been quantified (Hunt and Smith 2004). Paediatric valgo planus feet can be classified as flexible or rigid (Cass and Camasta 2010) and hypermobility in the foot is common but difficult to quantify.

Gait

The first steps during walking are controlled by the plantar support reflex and reflex gait. During a complete gait cycle, the centre of gravity is displaced twice on its vertical

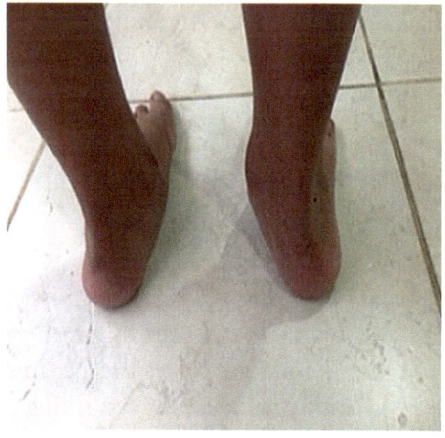

Fig. 5.2 Flat feet associated with hypermobility

axis (Perry 2005; Perry 2005a, b). The intermediate posture between the beginning of the equilibrium phase and the gait is when the centre of gravity starts to adjust itself for the first step (Neumann 2016). All muscles, even those in more distant muscle chains, are supportive of the gait process. Furthermore, the psychosocial state of an individual can alter the gait (Perry 2005; Perry 2005a, b).

Hypermobile individuals have gait impairments that add to impaired proprioception (Clayton et al. 2013, 2015) and leads to an abnormal and non-physiological gait pattern, with a consequent increased frequency of falls (Galli et al. 2011; Rombaut et al. 2011a, b).

References

Abrantes JMCS. Biomecânica da estabilidade articular. Rev Bras Educ Fis Esp. 2006;5:87–90.

Amadio AC, Costa PHL, Sacco ICN, Serrão JC, Araujo RC, Mochizuki L, et al. Introdução à Biomecânica para análise do movimento humano: descrição e aplicação dos métodos de medição. Rev Bras Fisiot. 1999;3:41–54.

Beighton P, Grahame R, Bird HA. Hypermobility of joints. 4th ed. London: Springer; 2012.

Bird HA. Joint and tissue laxity. In: Wright V, editor. Topical reviews of the rheumatic disorders. 2nd ed. Bristol: John Wright & Sons; 1983. p. 133–66.

Bird H, Knight I. Joint hypermobility in musicians. Infosheet #8. West Music School; 2012.

Bradley M, O'Donnell P. Atlas de anatomia: ultra-sonografia musculoesqueletica. Rio de Janeiro: Thieme Revienter; 2007.

Cass AD, Camasta CA. A review of tarsal coalition and pes planovalgus: clinical examination, diagnostic imaging, and surgical planning. J Foot Ankle Surg. 2010;49:274–93.

Chiodelli L, Pacheco AB, Missau TS, Silva AMT, Corrêa ECR. Influence of generalized joint hypermobility on temporomandibular joint, mastication and deglutition: a cross-sectional study. Rev CEFAC. 2015;17:890–8.

Clayton HA, Cressman EK, Henriques DYP. Proprioceptive sensitivity in EhlersDanlos syndrome patients. Exp Brain Res. 2013;230:311–21.

Clayton HA, Jones SAH, Henriques DYP. Proprioceptive precision is impaired in Ehlers-Danlos syndrome. Springerplus. 2015;4:1–8.

Dutton M. Guia de Sobrevivência do Fisioterapeuta: Manejando Condições Comuns. Porto Alegre: AMGH; 2012.

Enoka RM. Bases neuromecânicas da cinesiologia. 2. ed. São Paulo: Manole; 2000.

Ericson WB Jr, Wolman R. Orthopaedic management of the Ehlers-Danlos syndromes. Am J Med Genet C Semin Med Genet. 2017;175:188–94.

Fatoye FO, Mosaku SK, Komolafe MA, Eegunranti BA, Adebayo RA, Komolafe EO, et al. Depressive symptoms and associated factors following cerebrovascular accident among Nigerians. JMH. 2009;18:224–32.

Galli M, Cimolin V, Rigoldi C, Castori M, Celletti C, Albertini G, et al. Gait strategy in patients with Ehlers-Danlos syndrome hypermobility type: A kinematic and kinetic evaluation using 3D gait analysis. Res Dev Disabil. 2011;32:1663–8.

Hunt AE, Smith RM. Mechanics and control of the flat versus normal foot during the stance phase of walking. Clin Biomech (bristol, Avon). 2004;19:391–7.

Johns RJ, Wrigth V. Relative importance of various tissues in joint stiffness. J Appl Physiol. 1962; 17:824–828.

Kapandji AI. Fisiologia Articular: esquemas comentados de mecânica humana. São Paulo: Panamericana; Rio de Janeiro: Guanabara Koogan; 2000.

Kassel G. What's the difference between mobility vs. flexibility? 2018; https://barbend.com/mobility-vs-flexibility/.

Kendal FP, McCreary EK, Provance PG, Rodgers MC, Romani WA. Músculos: provas e funções. 5ª ed. Barueri: Manole; 2007. p. 3–47.

Kerr A, Macmillan CE, Uttley WS, Luqmani RA. Physiotherapy for children with hypermobility syndrome. Physiotherapy. 2000;86:313–7.

Kłodowski A, Rantalainen T. Multibody approach to musculoskeletal and joint loading. Arch Computat Methods Eng. 2015;22:237–67.

Levangie PK, Norkin CC. Joint structure and function: a comprehensive analysis. 5th ed. Philadelphia: F. A. Davis Company; 2011.

Lu TW, Chang CF. Biomechanics of human movement and its clinical applications. Kaohsiung J Med Sci. 2012;28(2 Suppl):S13–25.

Malina RM, Martinho DV, Santos JV, Silva MJC, Kozieł SM. Growth and maturity status of female soccer players: a narrative review. Int J Environ Res Public Health. 2021;18:1448.

Malina RM, Bouchard C. Growth, maturation, and physical activity. Champaign: Human Kinetics; 1991. p. 11–20.

Marino LHC, Lamari N, Marino NW Jr. Hipermobilidade articular nos joelhos da criança. Arq Ciênc Saúde. 2004;11:124–7.

Mekhael M, Labaki C, Bizdikian AJ, Bakouny Z, Otayek J, Yared F, et al. How do skeletal and postural parameters contribute to maintain balance during walking? Hum Mov Sci. 2020;72:1026582.

Mézières F. Originalité de la méthode Mézières. Paris: Maloine; 1984.

Myer GD, Ford KR, Paterno MV, Nick TG, Hewett TE. The effects of generalized joint laxity on risk of anterior cruciate ligament injury in young female athletes. Am J Sports Med. 2008;36:1073–80.

Neumann DA. Kinesiology of the musculoskeletal system: foundations for rehabilitation. 3rd ed. New York: Mosby; 2016.

Nordin M, Frankel V. Basic biomechanics of the skeletal system. 4th ed. Baltimore: Lippincot Willians & Wilkins; 2012.

Norkin CC, White J. Measurement of joint motion: a guide to goniometry. 5th ed. Philadelphia: F. A. Davis Company; 2017.

Perry J. Análise de Marcha—Marcha Normal. São Paulo: Manole; 2005a. vol 1.

Perry J. Análise de Marcha—Marcha Patológica. São Paulo: Manole; 2005b. vol 2.

Perry J. Análise de Marcha—Sistemas de Análise de Marcha. São Paulo: Manole; 2005. vol 3.

Pinheiro MB, Avelar BS, Teixeira-Salmela LF. Implicações clínicas das respostas dos tecidos musculares e conjuntivos ao estresse físico. Ter Man. 2013;11:111–6.

Purvis T. Mecânica articular II. Traduzido e Revisado por Malucelli MMF. Oklahoma: RTS, LLC; 2017.

Ramesh R, Von Arx O, Azzopardi T, Schranz PJ. The risk of anterior cruciate ligament rupture with generalised joint laxity. J Bone Joint Surg Br. 2005;87:800–3.

Rodrigues TL. Flexibilidade e alongamento. 20ª. Rio de Janeiro: Sprint; 1998.

Rombaut L, Malfait F, De Paepe A, Rimbaut S, Verbruggen G, De Wandele I, et al. Impairment and impact of pain in female patients with Ehlers-Danlos syndrome: a comparative study with fibromyalgia and rheumatoid arthritis. Arthritis Rheum. 2011a;63:1979–87.

Rombaut L, Malfait F, De Wandele I, Cools A, Thijs Y, De Paepe A, et al. Medication, surgery, and physiotherapy among patients with the hypermobility type of Ehlers-Danlos syndrome. Arch Phys Med Rehabil. 2011b;92:1106–12.

Steinmann B, Royce PM, Superti-Furga A. The Ehlers-Danlos syndrome. In: Royce PM, Steinmann B, editors. Connective tissue and its heritable disorders. New York: Wiley-Liss; 2003. p. 431–523.

Whiting WC, Zernicke RF. Biomechanics of musculoskeletal injury. 2nd ed. Champaign: Human Kinetics; 2008.

6

Mechanical Consequences of Joint Hypermobility

Trunk Instability

Trunk instability occurs due to several factors, including muscle deficit with decreased strength, hypotrophy, muscle weakness, and fatigue (Fig. 6.1). In addition to these influences, the weight of the trunk itself contributes to anterior tilt due to the lack of antigravitational musculature to keep the trunk erect, and to the weakness of the muscles that promote vertebral pelvic segmental stability (Moraes 2002). As for the most important core muscles of the lumbar region, it is believed that the inadequacies of the transversus spinalis, erector of the spine, quadratus lumborum, and latissimus dorsi may also cause the failure of stabilization of the trunk (Winter 2009). In turn, this process can cause a hypermobile individual to sit with the trunk bent forwards.

Spinal stability is dependent upon static elements, such as ligaments and bones, together with the dynamic

© The Author(s), under exclusive license to Springer Nature Switzerland AG 2023
N. Lamari and P. Beighton, *Hypermobility in Medical Practice*,
In Clinical Practice, https://doi.org/10.1007/978-3-031-34914-0_6

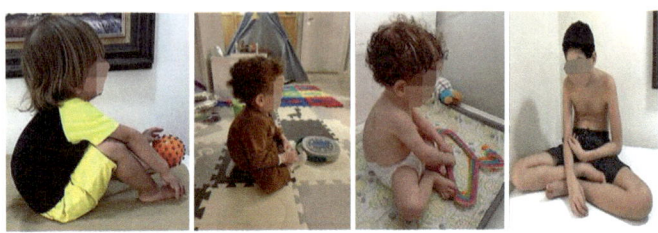

Fig. 6.1 Children with JH sitting with trunk stabilization failure due to soft tissue inefficiency

maintenance of each vertebral body and abdominal muscles. Weakness of the anterior abdominal muscles allows the pelvis to tilt forward. In these circumstances, these muscles are unable to exert upward traction on the pelvis, which is necessary for maintaining a good alignment. For these reasons, affected individuals mostly sit in a concave position. This spinal malalignment is a primary cause of vertebral pathologies such as disc degeneration, osteoarthrosis and spondylolisthesis, amongst others. Pain is a frequent consequence which may cause considerable distress (Mekhael et al. 2020).

Anterior Trunk Hyperflexion

Anterior hyperflexion of the trunk, with the hands flat on the ground and the knees extended, is achieved by the anterior flexion of the vertebral column and hips (Norkin and White 1997). It can have mechanical repercussions with hyperdistension of the entire posterior muscle chain, and cause possible vertebral instability. In the spine, an increase in the posterior intervertebral space, sagging of the posterior longitudinal ligament can lead to posterior displacement of the disc. This condition may lead to the disc protrusion with consequent nerve root compression and posterior vertebral listhesis (retrolisthesis) may follow. With aging a gradual decrease in the antigravity musculature strength that leads to undesirable postures to achieve body realignment. The pelvis may tilt anteriorly, further forcing hyperextension. Increased distensibility of the posterior thigh muscles (knee flexors) causes a decrease in strength that leads to knee hyperextension (Kapandji 2000).

Rotation of the Lower Limbs

For individuals with JH, there is a tendency to ambulate with rotation of the lower limbs (Fig. 6.2). This is predominantly an internal rotation, in which the capsular ligaments of the hip are distended, causing instability and anteversion of the femoral head. This process rotates the

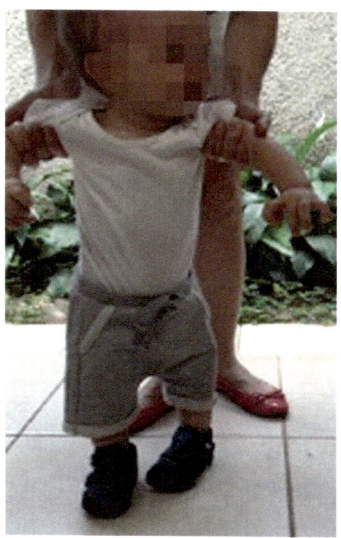

Fig. 6.2 Internal deviation of the lower limb of a child with JH while walking

femur internally, with deviation of the limb axis. Moreover, there is an alteration in the physiological valgus of the knee and, for greater stability, the limb rotates internally and cannot return to the normal position. Compensation occurs with the hyperdistensibility of the knee capsule ligament, which also leads to a disarray of internal structures. The resultant pain further increases the deviation. In this way, there is compensation of the limb alignment with respect to axial load (Whiting and Zernicke 2008).

Asymmetric rotational changes can be femoral torsion (rotation) and internal or external tibial torsion. External tibial torsion often occurs with growth, ranging from 0° at birth to 20° in adults. Internal torsion is common at birth and may or may not resolve with growth. Children with internal torsion may regularly sit in a "W" position or sleep in pronation with the legs extended or flexed and internally rotated. These children assume this position possibly because they feel more comfortable (Whiting 2009).

In the context of biomechanical adaptation, the tibia rotates internally, deviating the foot medially and in pronation. Consequently, there is a greater displacement of the body weight on the medial border of the foot. Collapse of the longitudinal plantar arch leads to the flat-foot deformity. In plantar arch collapse there is generalized hypotonia of the ligaments, with intrinsic muscle weakness of the foot and plantar fascia. In this situation, there is a lack of sufficient tension to maintain the plantar arch (Norkin and White 2017).

Digital Hyperextension

Intrinsic muscles of the hand tense in order to stabilize structures which are unstable due to ligament laxity. This situation causes incorrect positioning of the finger joints,

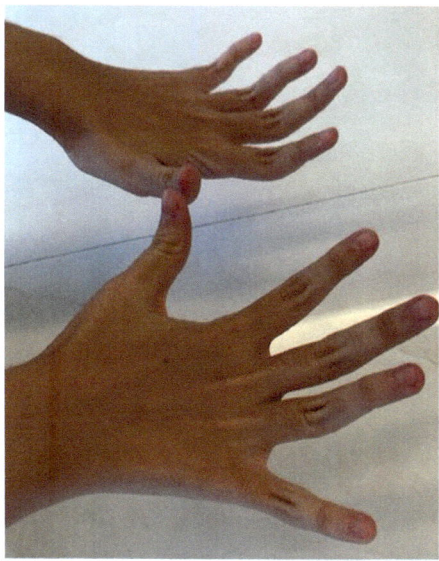

Fig. 6.3 Hypermobility in finger joints with compensatory hyperextension

leading to compensatory hyperextension (Fig. 6.3). Muscle tension, which consists of the contraction of a muscle in the performance of tasks, can become excessive and hinder its disposition, which is often inevitable in the hands of some individuals with hypermobility. This excessive muscle tension, besides being limiting sobre a and painful, especially if it persists for long periods, can affect other tissues, resulting in inflammation, tendinitis, or overuse syndrome (Dutton 2012).

Instability and Dislocation of the Knee

Mechanical considerations of knee injuries are relevant to the understanding of the frequent episodes of instabilities or dislocations in hypermobile individuals (Fig. 6.4). An

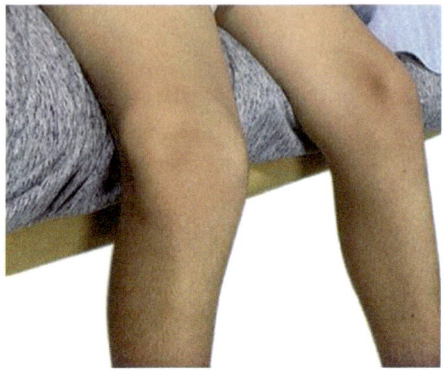

Fig. 6.4 Patellar dislocation in a child with hypermobility in the knees

anatomical factor that predisposes an individual to patel-lofemoral dislocation is an abnormal Q angle. The Q angle is a deviation between the line of traction of the quadri-ceps of the thigh and patellar ligament. It is usually meas-ured as the angle between a line from the anterosuperior iliac spine to the centre of the patella and a line from cen-tre of the patella to the anterior tibial tuberosity. The Q angle of 10° is considered normal. Larger angles may result in lateral patellar dislocations when quadriceps contraction reduces the angle. Tibiofemoral dislocation is more severe and less common. Meniscus injury is usually simultane-ous with ligament sprain and there are differences in the mechanisms of injury to the medial and lateral menisci (Trilha Junior et al. 2009).

Knee sprains result from movements that exceed normal limits of the joint. When forced beyond this natural restric-tion, the ligaments can be subjected to a strain greater than their elastic limit, placing them in the plastic region of their load-extension curve. The result is a permanent deformation of the ligaments and the magnitude of defor-mation depends on the force applied. Knee ligament sprain can occur in any direction of motion. The most common form of injury occurs when the foot is fixed and the femur rotates medially with reference to the tibia, which at the same time rotates laterally (Trilha Junior et al. 2009).

Flat Feet

The term flat feet refers to a reduction of the plantar arch and is associated with a talus valgus, which causes medial rotation of the tibial and femoral axes. In this situation, there is a tendency towards a valgus knee, which directs the patellae towards the medial direction (Peterson 2002).

Flatfoot may be congenital or acquired. The congenital flatfoot has laxity of ligaments, with hypermobile medio-tarsal and subtalar joints and a short calcaneal tendon. The acquired flatfoot results from muscular, postural, or static imbalance, excessive weight, muscle fatigue, use of inappropriate footwear, and bad walking habits. Flatfoot may arise if there is an increased load on the lower extremities as a whole. The condition results in increased internal rotation of the leg, shifting support to the medial border of the foot, with a consequent reduction of the plantar arch due to lack of ligament support and hyperdistensibility of the plantar fascia. Laxity of the plantar and medial ligaments leads to eversion of the calcaneus and shortening of the lateral and peroneal ligaments (Hunt and Smith 2004).

It is well established that the tibialis anterior muscle plays no role in normal static support of the longitudinal arch of the foot. During conditions with dynamic loads, however, muscle contraction assists the osteoligamentous structures, which are the primary source of arch support. Moreover, individuals with flat feet require muscular support of the arches, especially by the anterior tibial muscle. Collagen deficiency makes ligaments more friable and

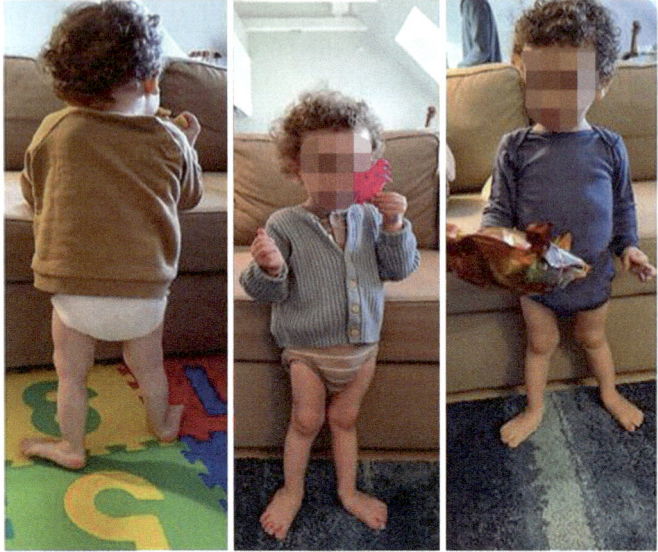

Fig. 6.5 Collapse of the plantar arch in children due to lack of ligament and plantar fascia tension, with a decrease in the intrinsic musculature strength of the foot

less likely to reach the maximum tension required to promote the stability of bones that compose the plantar arch. Maintenance of this arch becomes untenable if there is a lack of ligament tension and plantar fascia. Similarly, a decrease in the strength of the intrinsic muscles that leads to the collapse of the plantar arch, thereby producing the flattening of the feet (Fig. 6.5) (Hunt and Smith 2004).

References

Dutton M. Guia de Sobrevivência do Fisioterapeuta: Manejando Condições Comuns. Porto Alegre: AMGH; 2012.

Hunt AE, Smith RM. Mechanics and control of the flat versus normal foot during the stance phase of walking. Clin Biomech (Bristol, Avon). 2004;19:391–7.

Kapandji AI. Fisiologia Articular: esquemas comentados de mecânica humana. São Paulo: Panamericana; Rio de Janeiro: Guanabara Koogan; 2000.

Mekhael M, Labaki C, Bizdikian AJ, Bakouny Z, Otayek J, Yared F, et al. How do skeletal and postural parameters contribute to maintain balance during walking? Hum Mov Sci. 2020;72:1026582.

Moraes LFS. Os princípios das cadeias musculares na avaliação dos desconfortos corporais e constrangimentos posturais em motoristas do transporte coletivo [dissertação]. Florianópolis: Universidade Federal de Santa Catarina; 2002.

Norkin CC, White J. Medida do movimento articular: Manual de goniometria. 2ª ed. Porto Alegre: Artes Medicas; 1997. p. 217–32.

Norkin CC, White J. Measurement of joint motion: a guide to goniometry. 5th ed. Philadelphia: F. A. Davis Company; 2017.

Peterson L. Lesões do esporte: prevenção e tratamento. 3ª ed. Barueri, SP: Manole; 2002.

Trilha Junior M, Fancello EA, Roesler CRM, More ADO. Three-dimensional numerical simulation of human knee joint mechanics. Acta Ortop Bras. 2009;17:18–23.

Whiting WC. Biomecanica functional e das lesões musculoesqueléticas. Rio de Janeiro: Guanabara Koogan; 2009.

Whiting WC, Zernicke RF. Biomechanics of Musculoskeletal Injury. 2nd ed. Champaign: Human Kinetics; 2008.

Winter DA. Biomechanics and motor control of human movement. 4th ed. Hoboken: Wiley; 2009.

7

Ehlers-Danlos Syndromes

Background and Classification of the Ehlers-Danlos Syndromes

The fields of medical genetics, rheumatology and other specialities have made numerous contributions to the historical understanding and the evolution of concepts related to the nomenclature and nosology of hypermobile Ehlers-Danlos syndrome and hypermobility syndrome. In this context, a book by Peter Beighton, "The Ehlers-Danlos syndrome" (1970) (Beighton 1970) and another by Beighton, Grahame and Bird "Hypermobility of Joints" (1983) (Beighton et al. 1983) are relevant.

In successive editions of his magisterial monograph "Heritable Disorders of Connective Tissue", McKusick (1956) offered important historical data pertaining to the Ehlers-Danlos syndrome (EDS). He traced the history of the syndrome and emphasized that no other hereditary

© The Author(s), under exclusive license to Springer Nature Switzerland AG 2023
N. Lamari and P. Beighton, *Hypermobility in Medical Practice*, In Clinical Practice, https://doi.org/10.1007/978-3-031-34914-0_7

connective tissue disorder, except possibly osteogenesis imperfecta, has a history as old as that of EDS. He stated that the first case was described in 1682 by Amsterdam surgeon Job van Meekeren. Simmonds and Keer (2007) report that hyperextension of the metacarpal joints, hyper-flexion of the feet and hyperlordosis was depicted by Peter Rubens in his painting "The Three Graces" (1638–1640), which is displayed in the Prado Museum in Madrid. Similarly, the musical successes of Paganini in the nineteenth Century were attributed to the extreme mobility of his hands.

In 1956, McKusick (1956) mentioned that several dermatologists, including Kopp in 1888 and Williams in 1892, had published sparse references to this condition, which was regarded as a curiosity in the "rubber men of India". Kopp's report was noteworthy for having described the condition in a father and son, thereby recognising the possible familial nature of the disorder. In 1888, Gould and Pyle published a photograph taken in Budapest of a sideshow exhibitionist named Felix Wehrle, "who, besides having the power to stretch his skin, could easily bend his fingers backwards and forwards". The photograph taken in 1880 is the first known photographic documentation of an individual with EDS, which is also mentioned in the book by Gould and Pyle (1897) "Anomalies and Curiosities of Medicine" (Hamonet et al. 2016). In Unna's laboratory in Hamburg, Du Mesnil (1890), Williams (1892) and Unna (1894) published accounts of histological studies of the syndrome. In 1901, Ehlers reported joint looseness associated with a proneness to subcutaneous haemorrhage. In 1908, Danlos completed the clinical description with the inclusion of pseudo-tumours developed in subcutaneous sites.

In a 2016 review of the history of Ehlers-Danlos syndrome (Hamonet et al. 2016) focuses on the Russian dermatologist Tschernogobow. The authors stated that the concomitant manifestations of skin hyperextensibility and joint hypermobility in EDS was first described by Tschernogobow (Russia, 1891), Ehlers (Denmark, 1898) and Danlos (France, 1908), who introduced concepts that have marked the history of the syndrome to this day. Alexandre Nicolaiev Tschernogobow (also written as Chernogobov or Csernogobov) presented the cases of two patients to the Dermatology and Venereology Society in Moscow. The first was a 17-year-old who had repeated joint dislocations, nodules on the skin, brittle skin and hyperextensibility, multiple scars resulting from trivial trauma, poor wound healing and pseudo-tumours on the knees, elbows and other parts of the body, which Tschernogobow attributed to a connective tissue disorder. The second patient was a 57-year-old man who had undergone operations for several tumours and had severe healing problems (Parapia and Jackson 2008) In 1900, Sir Malcolm Morris presented a case to the London Dermatology Society (Weber 1936).

The syndrome was originally described by Edvard Ehlers in 1898 in Denmark and Henri-Alexandre Danlos in 1908 in Paris. Both authors published individual case studies in which the common factor was ligament laxity leading to joint hypermobility and hyperextensibility of the skin. In 1900, Edvard Lauritz Ehlers made the first complete description of EDS to physicians of the Danish Dermatology Society in Copenhagen, presenting the case of a 21-year-old law student. The presentation was entitled "*Cutis laxa*". Besides hypermobility, Ehlers also described a large part of the currently known clinical manifestations of EDS, such as bleeding, brittle skin, joint dislocations and dysautonomia, and suggested the hereditary nature of the syndrome by stating that the patient's father had different joint manifestations.

In 1908, the French dermatologist Henri Alexandre Danlos presented a patient with EDS under the title of *cutis laxa* to the French Dermatology Society in Paris. This individual had loose skin over his elbows and knees which resulted from hematomas. Danlos emphasised that the elbows and knees were affected and he highlighted that the skin was thin and could be stretched extensively. The term "cutis laxa" pertains to gross skin laxity, which may be secondary, as in this case described by Danlos, or exist in isolation as an autonomous condition. The emphasis placed on the hyperextended skin led to negative consequences on part of physicians regarding this syndrome at the time, as many discarded the diagnosis in the absence of "extraordinary stretching" of the skin. It is now known that stretching of the skin can be moderate and even absent in certain types of EDS (Hamonet et al. 2016). Weber (1936) made a considerable historical contribution by reporting six examples in England, the first of which was a boy presented by Sir Malcolm Morris to the London Dermatology Society in 1900, even though the diagnosis was not conclusive (Cohn 1907). Beighton saw this patient again around 1970 and confirmed that Morris' diagnosis of EDS was correct. Weber (1936) outlined these conditions, highlighting hyperextensibility and brittleness of the skin, as well as joint looseness in his patients, stating that the eponymous terminology of Ehlers-Danlos syndrome was appropriate for this condition.

In this historical sequence, Hamonet et al. (2016) reported that Schulmann and Levy Coblentz (1932) associated the two names, "Ehlers and Danlos". Thereafter, Achille Miget (1933) used this format in a thesis. The use of this conjoined eponym was formalised in 1936 by Frederick Parkes-Weber and this style has been maintained ever since (Weber 1936). Throughout his life, Parkes-Weber was a legendary scholar of rare diseases. He was the doyen of British syndrome diagnosticians and his name is associated with several uncommon disorders.

There is now extensive and unprecedented knowledge on various biochemical and genetic aspects of the different types of EDS. Manifestations of the syndrome are still often considered to be a curiosity due to the very elastic skin and the fact that joint hypermobility recalls notions of deformation. However, despite these advances, Job van Meek'ren is known to have made the first partial description of the syndrome (Hamonet et al. 2016) and the description made by Tschernogobow in 1891 continues to be one of the best descriptions of EDS in the literature (Grahame 2016).

Historically, hypermobility, which is a striking characteristic of EDS, was associated with other manifestations or joint deformities. Joint hypermobility as a cause of pain and recurring joint effusion was first cited by Sutro (1947) who described 13 young adults with pain and effusion in the knees and ankles developing during a military training course. Subsequently, Massie and Howorth (1951) recognised the aetiological importance of generalised joint laxity in the pathogenesis of congenital hip dislocation. Carter and Sweetnam (1958) associated recurring knee and shoulder sub-luxation to congenital hip dislocation. Hass and Hass (1958) reported foot posture deformities, scoliosis, hip and elbow luxation in five children and recognised joint hypermobility without the presence of skin abnormalities as an independent articular disorder in the general EDS category. Callegarini (1957) and Levine (1958) associated hyperextensibility of the finger joints rheumatic fever in children. Carter and Wilkinson (1964) demonstrated a close association with family joint laxity. McKusick (1966) reported that generalised joint looseness is also characteristic of hereditary connective tissue disorders including Marfan syndrome, Ehlers-Danlos syndrome and osteogenesis imperfecta.

Joint hypermobility, which is a striking characteristic of hypermobile EDS, appeared for the first time as an important clinical entity in the rheumatological literature in 1967. This recognition occurred when Kirk et al. (1967) described a joint hypermobility syndrome characterised by musculoskeletal symptoms in the presence of generalised joint laxity of a benign nature in normal individuals. These authors also emphasised the overlapping of this syndrome with hereditary connective tissue disorders.

Medical geneticist Peter Beighton has made diverse contributions to hypermobility and EDS, including the Beighton Method for quantifying the magnitude of joint hypermobility. This approach was scientifically validated in 1973 (Beighton et al. 1973) and is employed in both clinical practice and research. A numerical score derived from this method was developed during an epidemiological investigation in Africa. and remains among the current criteria for the diagnosis of EDS (Malfait et al. 2017).

A historical review of EDS by Parapia and Jackson (2008) highlights Beighton's contributions in 1970 in his first book entitled "The Ehlers-Danlos Syndrome". Beighton commented on one of these individuals with EDS that were presented to the Dermatological Society of Denmark in 1899. One of the cases had delayed walking and frequent subluxation of the knees. Another was identified by French physician Henri-Alexandre Danlos (1844–1912). Other isolated case reports appeared in the first half of the twentieth Century including those made by Tobias (1934) Ronchese (1936) and McKusick (1972). The patients' manifestations extended from mild symptoms consisting of simply a tendency toward becoming injured easily to more severe problems such as formation of hematomas and bleeding of the nose, intestine, lungs and urinary tract.

The formal classification of EDS began at the end of the 1960s (Beighton 1970; Mckusick 1972). The Berlin

Nosology (Beighton et al. 1988) published in 1988 presented diagnostic criteria for the main connective tissue-related disorders, including EDS. In this period, the syndrome became better understood, with greater recognition of its multisystemic nature. One of the difficulties encountered at the time was the lack of valid criteria for the diagnosis of the syndrome (Grahame et al. 2000).

Beighton and colleagues went on to write several other books related to hypermobility and EDS, including Beighton et al. (1983, 1989, 1999, 2012). Greta Beighton, Peter's wife, was a co-author in Beighton and Beighton (1986) and Beighton and Beighton (1997). Subsequently, book chapters (Beighton 1992a, b) and scientific articles appeared.

Beighton's scientific publications with an emphasis on EDS began in 1968, when he presented an article on the lethal complications of EDS (Beighton 1968a). In 1969, he wrote about the orthopedic aspects of the syndrome (Beighton and Horan 1969) addressed surgical aspects (Beighton and Horan 1969; Beighton and Bull 1970; Beighton et al. 1970) and delineated a possible subtype of EDS, Marfanoid Hypermobility Syndrome (Walker et al. 1969). He also wrote about calcification of breast tissue in the Ehlers-Danlos syndrome (Tapley and Beighton 2009).

Beighton made considerable contributions regarding the manifestations of EDS on the skin (Grahame and Beighton 1969, 1971; Beighton 1971b, 1972a, 1973, 1974; Goldblatt et al. 1988) as well as other studies on the beginning of connective tissue disorders (Beighton 1972b, c). He also highlighted the familial nature of hypermobility (Beighton and Horan 1970) and made many other contributions specifically to the study of EDS (Beighton and Wells 1968; Beighton 1968b, 1969, 1971a, 1977; Beighton et al. 1969; Beighton and Curtis 1985; Viljoen et al. 1987; Maeland et al. 2011; Wandele et al. 2013).

In the 1960s, Beighton was already addressing subjects that are found in the current literature, such as the gastrointestinal (Beighton et al. 1969; Korterink et al. 2014; Fikree et al. 2015; Pacey et al. 2015) obstetric (Volkov et al. 2007; Castori et al. 2012) cardiological (Atzinger et al. 2011; Mathias et al. 2011; Delling and Vasan 2014; Kozanoglu et al. 2016; Hakim et al. 2017a) orthopaedic (Tobias et al. 2013; Czaprowski 2014; Connelly et al. 2015; Stern et al. 2016; ; Ericson and Wolman 2017) and ophthalmological manifestations of the syndrome (Rose et al. 2008; Gharbiya et al. 2012).

In 1997, in Villefranche-sur-Mer, France, Beighton proposed a new Nosology that classified EDS into six subtypes, in which joint hypermobility syndrome became recognised as Ehlers-Danlos syndrome hypermobility type (Beighton et al. 1997). In the last two decades, this Villefranche Nosology has been widely used as the standard for clinical diagnosis of the subtypes of EDS. In most of these conditions, mutations have now been identified in collagen coding genes or genes that code collagen-modifying enzymes.

In 1999, Beighton received an international research award from the Ehlers-Danlos Foundation in the USA.

In 2000, Grahame et al. (2000) proposed a complete spectrum of new subtypes of EDS with mutations which had been identified in a newly recognised set of genes. However, difficulties remained due to the overlapping characteristics of the types listed by the Nosology and it was suggested in this study that there was a need for an international consensus.

In 2017, the International Consortium on Ehlers-Danlos Syndrome and Related Disorders proposed a classification that recognises 13 subtypes, with clinical criteria for each subtype (Fig. 7.1). There is vast genetic heterogeneity and phenotypic variability in the subtypes of EDS, as well as the clinical overlap among the types and other hereditary connective tissue disorders. In this consortium, the Ehlers-Danlos syndrome hypermobility type received a new denomination: "hypermobile Ehlers-Danlos syndrome" (hEDS). The definitive diagnosis of all subtypes, except hEDS, is now based on molecular confirmation with identification of the causal genetic variant(s) of hypermobility disorders (Malfait et al. 2017). The consortium also maintained the Beighton method among its diagnostic criteria, but with considerations by age group and body location and the inclusion of the five-point questionnaire proposed by Hakim and Grahame (2003). Lamari et al. (2022) suggest the inclusion of other variables to characterize JH in clinical practice.

Historically, hEDS has received several designations including the joint hypermobility syndrome, Ehlers-Danlos syndrome hypermobility type and EDS type III. In the current nosology, hypermobile EDS is considered to be the most common form of EDS (Malfait et al. 2017).

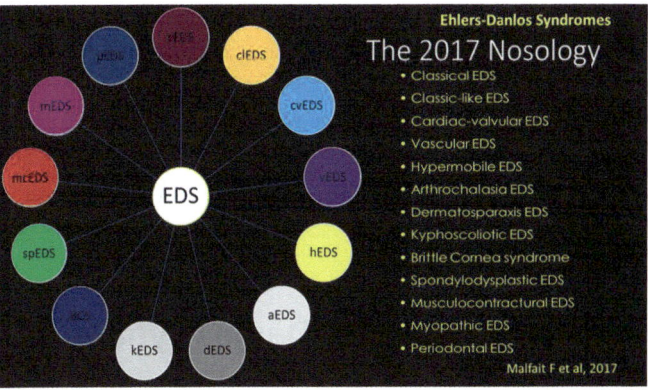

Fig. 7.1 Illustration of subtypes of Ehlers-Danlos syndromes presented in the 2017 Nosology (Malfait et al. 2017) (Mateus Lamari's doctoral thesis, 2021)

The new 2017 Nosology (Malfait et al. 2017) has made contributions for geneticists and difficulties for clinicians with more robust criteria for hEDS. Also in 2017, exclusion criteria were established for hEDS in the absence of other collagen disorders. In this way, hypermobility spectrum disorders prioritise musculoskeletal manifestations in the presence of joint hypermobility (Castori et al. 2017). It is now evident that these are the same conditions which were established by Kirk et al. (1967). Specifically, they refer to the original joint hypermobility syndrome, but now disregarding the benign nature of the disorder. This nomenclature overcomes enormous cultural difficulties, despite now emphasising the pathological issues.

The term "joint hypermobility syndrome" had been excluded in the Villefranche Nosology (Hakim and Grahame 2003) and is not mentioned in the 2017 Nosology (Malfait et al. 2017). It was proposed that "hypermobility spectrum disorders" be used for individuals with symptomatic joint hypermobility who do not meet the criteria for EDS or other syndromes. These constitute a clinically relevant group of conditions related to joint hypermobility and are used for the description and exclusion of diagnoses. They are distinguishable from hEDS and other syndromes with joint hypermobility due to the phenotypic domains of hypermobility spectrum disorders, which are generally limited to the musculoskeletal system by manifestations secondary to joint hypermobility (Castori et al. 2017).

Hypermobile Ehlers-Danlos Syndrome

Hypermobile EDS is an autosomal dominant hereditary disorder of the connective tissue with other patterns of heredity presents in some families (Castori et al. 2017). It is a heterogeneous genetic disorder (Hakim and Grahame 2004; Korterink et al. 2014) that affects the formation of collagen, with a small number of cases reported due to the haploinsufficiency of tenascin X (Zweers et al. 2003). The genetic determinants of hEDS are presumed to be abnormalities of collagen (Malfait et al. 2010) with pleiotropic manifestations in the condition. In this condition, a single gene controls several features of the phenotype, with multiple effects that are often unrelated (Lastname, et al. 2022) but affect the quality of life of these patients (Malfait et al. 2020).

Hypermobile EDS is influenced by gender and occurs predominantly in females. It is also the only type of EDS with no confirmed cause (Wijnhoven et al. 2006). It predisposes affected individuals to musculoskeletal and extraskeletal conditions (Tobias et al. 2013; Ericson and Wolman 2017; Bulbena et al. 2017; Fikree et al. 2017a, b, Hakim et al. 2017a, b). This form of the EDS is multisystemic, with clinical variations that affect the skin, ligaments, joints, blood vessels and internal organs (Paepe and Malfait 2012). The abnormalities are primary musculoskeletal manifestations and there is sometimes pain, fatigue, sleep disorders, anxiety and a poor quality of life (Tinkle et al. 2017).

When considering that hEDS accounts for 80–90% of cases of EDS, the presumed prevalence is not less than 1/5000. A much higher frequency of 7.5/1000–20/1000 (0.75–2%) has been proposed for symptomatic generalised joint hypermobility, as approximately 10% of affected individuals develop related symptoms throughout life (Hakim and Sahota 2006).

Hypermobile EDS is the most common systemic hereditary disorder of the connective tissue in humans, with 10 million affected persons in the United Kingdom, 10 million in the USA, 17 million in Europe and 255 million around the world (Mulvey et al. 2013). Phenotypic expression is variable, even within families, which makes the diagnosis challenging (Paepe and Malfait 2012).

Diagnosis of Hypermobile Ehlers-Danlos Syndrome

The diagnosis of hEDS is clinical and based on widely accepted diagnostic criteria along with the exclusion of other partially overlapping hereditary connective tissue diseases. No instrumental, histopathological/ultrastructural or molecular finding is considered pathognomonic of hEDS and at present there is no sufficiently reliable laboratory test for confirmation of the diagnosis (Bravo 2009; Castori 2013).

In March 2017, the new Nosology (Malfait et al. 2017) used the denomination "hypermobile Ehlers-Danlos syndrome". This meets the broad criteria and the range of systemic manifestations associated with hypermobility (Malfait et al. 2017).

Clinical Manifestations in Hypermobility and Hypermobile EDS

Hypermobile EDS can have widespread systemic manifestations, some of which are benign, whereas others are potentially lethal. The signs and symptoms are classified as musculoskeletal and extra-skeletal (Beighton 1970; Bulbena et al. 2017; Ericson and Wolman 2017; Fikree et al. 2017a; Hakim et al. 2017b). Henkel and Strides (2010) cites a study addressing the main clinical manifestations, such as musculoskeletal tissue flaccidity, noninflammatory pain in the joints and spinal column, joint dislocations, soft tissue injuries, problems with support structures, such as the pelvic floor, pain amplification syndrome, psychosocial manifestations, anxiety, depression, obesity, isolation and anger. The latter is often directed at physicians who are not able to help the patient.

Other studies report problems associated with joint hypermobility and hEDS, such as pain, fatigue, headache, scoliosis, flat feet, hypotonia, proprioceptive dysfunction, haemorrhagic syndrome, dysautonomia and dystonia, as well as digestive, bladder-sphincter, respiratory, dental, otorhinolaryngological, ophthalmological, gynaecological, obstetric and cognitive disorders, among other manifestations that are encountered in daily clinical practice (Mintz-Itkin et al. 2009; Mack 2010; Hamonet 2013; Fikree et al. 2015; Landry et al. 2015; Stern et al. 2016). Anxiety, depression, schizophrenia and neurological developmental disorders, such as attention deficit, hyperactivity and dyspraxia, are among the other clinical manifestations that are also occasionally associated with joint hypermobility (Baeza-Velasco et al. 2015; Bulbena et al. 2015).

Children with hEDS/HSD can develop problems as a result of increased joint mobility, which begin with pain (Adib et al. 2005; Kemp et al. 2010; Scheper et al. 2016). Reported problems are proprioception deficit (Fatoye et al. 2009a; Schubert-Hjalmarsson et al. 2012) joint instability (Beighton et al. 1969) joint luxation and subluxation, nerve pain (Daniels et al. 2016) extra-articular factors (Hakim and Grahame 2004; Kirby and Davies 2007) psychological symptoms (Beighton et al. 1969; Pacey et al. 2013) an abnormal gait pattern, impairment of physical fitness (Kirby et al. 2005; Kirby and Davies 2007; Falkerslev et al. 2013) and limitations in recreational activities (Jansson et al. 2004; Schubert-Hjalmarsson et al. 2012; Birt et al. 2014).

The skin of affected individuals with EDS differs from normal skin. The texture is soft, silky or velvety to the touch, hyperextensible and may be transparent (Malfait et al. 2010) In addition, the skin is fragile and healing may be compromised with atrophied striae (Burcharth and Rosenberg 2012; Jacks and Zirwas 2016) Hernias (Nelson et al. 2015) or weakness of the pelvic floor may also develop (Tinkle 2010).

Cardiovascular manifestations have been reported, with a 28–67% frequency of mitral valve prolapse in patients with hEDS (Dolan et al. 1997; McDonnell et al. 2006; Mathias et al. 2011; Delling and Vasan 2014; Kozanoglu et al. 2016). Orthostatic postural tachycardia syndrome, chronic fatigue syndrome, orthostatic intolerance (Rowe et al. 1999; Gazit et al. 2003; Hakim et al. 2017a) symptoms of systemic dysautonomia (Hakim and Grahame 2004; Eccles et al. 2015) and sympathetic neurogenic dysfunction (Wandele et al. 2014) are also reported.

Gastrointestinal involvement in the hEDS may comprise functional and morphological manifestations. (Wandele et al. 2013) Debilitating constipation in individuals with hEDS can occur at any age (Korterink et al. 2014; Scheper et al. 2016; Fikree et al. 2017b). Urinary incontinence and urinary tract infection are also found in this population (McIntosh et al. 1995; Kort et al. 2003; Arunkalaivanan et al. 2009; Tinkle 2010; Castori et al. 2010a; Beiraghdar et al. 2013; Derpapas et al. 2015).

Psychological dysfunction and emotional problems, such as depression, anxiety, affective disorder, low self-confidence, negative thoughts, hopelessness and despair are common in people with EDS (Hagberg et al. 2004; Zarate et al. 2010; Castori et al. 2010b; Baeza-Velasco et al. 2011; Branson et al. 2011; Rombaut et al. 2011a; Berglund et al. 2015; Sinibaldi et al. 2015; Hershenfeld et al. 2016).

Temporomandibular hypermobility and instability may occur, even in children (Adair and Hecht 1993). Local pain, luxation, bruxism (Sipilä et al. 2011; Nosouhian et al. 2015) periodontitis (Rahman et al. 2003) and difficulty with anaesthesia during dental procedures have been reported (Arendt-Nielsen et al. 1990; Hakim et al. 2005). In teeth, altered morphology, hypoplasia of the enamel and tooth fractures may be a feature (Coster et al. 2005a, b).

Neurological manifestations sometimes occur in children with hypermobility. These include developmental coordination disorder, poor fine and gross motor skills (Adib et al. 2005; Pacey et al. 2013) attention deficit, hyperactivity and dyspraxia (Baeza-Velasco et al. 2015; Bulbena et al. 2015). Fatigue, dizziness, fainting, syncope, memory and concentration problems (Wandele et al. 2014) and, especially, headache in individuals with hEDS have been noted (Jacome 1999; Rozen et al. 2006; Milhorat et al. 2007; Murray et al. 2013; Wandele et al. 2013; Easton et al. 2014; Neilson and Martin 2014; Castori et al. 2015; Hamonet et al. 2015).

Musculoskeletal complaints in hEDS manifest as joint pain of a non-inflammatory origin and/or spinal pain, with joint instability and consequent luxation or subluxation in peripheral joints as well as central joints. These conditions include temporomandibular, sacroiliac and hip joints, and there is a high potential for disability (Czaprowski 2014; Gazit et al. 2016).

Orthopaedic manifestations are commonly found in patients with hEDS, notably postural kyphosis (el-Shahaly and el-Sherif AK 1991; Tobias et al. 2013) scoliosis (Ainsworth and Aulicino 1993; Stanitski et al. 2000; Adib et al. 2005; Connelly et al. 2015; Stern et al. 2016) flat feet (Berglund et al. 2005; Evans and Rome 2011; Ross et al. 2011; Rigoldi et al. 2012) hyperextension of the knees (Marino et al. 2004) joint pain (Mallik et al. 1994;

Adib et al. 2005; Fatoye et al. 2009b) and nerve pain (Shirley et al. 2012; Daniels et al. 2016). Joint laxity can exert a negative impact on the physical health of affected children (Mallik et al. 1994; Everman and Robin 1998; Kerr et al. 2000; Ramesh et al. 2005; Myer et al. 2008) and can be followed by consequent degenerative processes (Simpson 2006) loss of muscle strength and endurance, and a reduction in the quality of life (Landry et al. 2015).

Complaints of pain are common among individuals with a diagnosis of hEDS (Jacome 1999; Murray et al. 2013; Wandele et al. 2013; Hamonet et al. 2015) the chronic nature of which has negative consequences for quality of life (Baeza-Velasco et al. 2011). Headaches are frequent, vary in both type and severity (Jacome 1999; Rozen et al. 2006; Milhorat et al. 2007; Murray et al. 2013; Neilson and Martin 2014; Castori et al. 2015) and contribute to disability in affected individuals (Rombaut et al. 2010a, b, 2011a, b, 2012a, b). Voermans et al. (2010) report that pain is common, severe and associated with functional impairment. The clinical presentation of joint hypermobility and pain varies in children (Landry et al. 2015) and pain is described in the entire body beginning in early childhood (Hamonet 2013).

Fatigue in hEDS has a multifactor aetiology and is found in most individuals with the condition. Fatigue involves a persistent sensation of weariness, a lack of energy and the sensation of exhaustion, with a negative impact on concentration (Castori et al. 2012). Contributing factors are pain, sleep disorders, dysautonomia, medications and allergies (Beighton et al. 1969; Sparto et al. 1997; Dickin and Doan 2008; Castori et al. 2011; Voermans et al. 2011; Ali Zekry et al. 2013; Scheper et al. 2013; Ericson and Wolman 2017; Hakim et al. 2017b;).

Individuals with hEDS report problems sleeping, such as insomnia and non-restoring sleep (Hakim and Grahame

2004; Dickin and Doan 2008; Murray et al. 2013) Other factors also affect the sleep quality of these individuals, such as pain, dysautonomia, poor sleep hygiene and medications (Voermans et al. 2010). Fibromyalgia is a common concomitant condition (Ofluoglu et al. 2006; Ting et al. 2012) and is strongly associated with sleep disorders, including abnormal sleep architecture (Dauvilliers and Touchon 2001; Besteiro González et al. 2011).

References

Adair SM, Hecht C. Association of generalized joint hypermobility with history, signs, and symptoms of temporomandibular joint dysfunction in children. Pediatr Dent. 1993;15:323–6.

Adib N, Davies K, Grahame R, Woo P, Murray KJ. Joint hypermobility syndrome in childhood. A not so benign multisystem disorder? Rheumatology (Oxford). 2005; 44:744–50.

Ainsworth SR, Aulicino PL. A survey of patients with Ehlers-Danlos syndrome. Clin Orthop Relat Res. 1993;286:250–6.

Ali Zekry O, Ali Ahmed M, Ali Elsayed Abd Elwahid H. The impact of fatigue on health related quality of life in adolescents with benign joint hypermobility syndrome. Egypt Rheumatol. 2013; 35:77–85.

Arendt-Nielsen L, Kaalund S, Bjerring P, Hogsaa B. Insufficient effect of local analgesics in Ehlers Danlos type III patients (connective tissue disorder). Acta Anaesthesiol Scand. 1990;34:358–61.

Arunkalaivanan AS, Morrison A, Jha S, Blann A. Prevalence of urinary and faecal incontinence among female members of the Hypermobility Syndrome Association (HMSA). J Obstet Gynaecol. 2009;29:126–8.

Atzinger CL, Meyer RA, Khoury PR, Gao Z, Tinkle BT. Cross-sectional and longitudinal assessment of aortic root dilation and valvular anomalies in hypermobile and classic Ehlers-Danlos syndrome. J Pediatr. 2011;158:826–30.

Baeza-Velasco C, Gély-Nargeot MC, Bulbena Vilarrasa A, Bravo JF. Joint hypermobility syndrome: problems that require psychological intervention. Rheumatol Int. 2011;31:1131–6.

Baeza-Velasco C, Pailhez G, Bulbena A, Baghdadli A. Joint hypermobility and the heritable disorders of connective tissue: clinical and empirical evidence of links with psychiatry. Gen Hosp Psychiatry. 2015;37(1):24–30.

Beighton P. Lethal complications of the Ehlers-Danlos syndrome. Br Med J. 1968a;3(656–9):34.

Beighton P. X-linked recessive inheritance in the Ehlers-Danlos syndrome. Br Med J. 1968b;3:409–11.

Beighton P. Ehlers-Danlos syndrome. Am J Dis Child. 1969;118:891.

Beighton P. The Ehlers-Danlos syndrome. London: William Heinemann Medical Books Ltd.; 1970.

Beighton P. Articular manifestations of the Ehlers-Danlos syndrome. Sem Arth Rheum. 1971a;3:246–61.

Beighton P. Cutis laxa. Clinical Delineation of Birth Defects. Part VII (8): 302–5: 1971b.

Beighton P. The dominant and recessive forms of cutis laxa. J Med Genet. 1972a;2:216–21.

Beighton P. The inherited disorders of connective tissue. Part I Bull Rheum Dis. 1972b;2:696–700.

Beighton P. The inherited disorders of connective tissue. Part II Bull Rheum Dis. 1972c;3:702–7.

Beighton P. Cutis laxa - a heterogeneous disorder. Birth Defects. 1974;10:126–31.

Beighton P. Clinical problems in the Ehlers-Danlos syndrome. Mod Med. 1977;2:2–5.

Beighton P, Beighton G. The man behind the syndrome. Heidelberg: Springer-Verlag; 1986.

Beighton P, Beighton G. The person behind the syndrome. Heidelberg: Springer-Verlag; 1997.

Beighton P, Bull JC. Plastic surgery in the Ehlers-Danlos syndrome. Plastic and Reconst Surg. 1970;45:606–9.

Beighton P, Curtis D. X-linked Ehlers-Danlos syndrome type V; the next generation. Clin Genet. 1985;27:472–8.

Beighton P, Horan F. Dominant inheritance in familial generalised articular hypermobility. J Bone Joint Surg. 1970;52B:145–7.

Beighton P, Lamont Murdoch J, Votteler T. Gastrointestinal complications of the Ehlers-Danlos syndrome. Gut. 1969;10:1004–8.

Beighton P, Bull JC, Edgerton MT. Plastic surgery in cutis laxa. Br J Plast Surg. 1970;23:285–90.

Beighton P, Solomon I, Soskolne L. Articular mobility in an African population. Ann Rheum Dis. 1973;32:413–8.

Beighton P, Grahame R, Bird H. Hypermobility of Joints. Heidelberg: Springer-Verlag; 1983.

Beighton P, de Paepe A, Danks D, Finidori G, Gedde-Dahl T, Goodman R, et al. International nosology of heritable disorders of connective tissue, Berlin, 1986. Am J Med Genet. 1988;29:581–94.

Beighton P, Grahame R, Bird H. Hypermobility of Joints. 2nd ed. Heidelberg: Springer-Verlag; 1989.

Beighton P, Grahame R, Bird H. Hypermobility of joints. 3rd ed. Heidelberg: Springer-Verlag; 1999.

Beighton P, Grahame R, Bird H. Hypermobility of joints. 4th ed. Heidelberg: Springer-Verlag; 2012.

Beighton P. The Ehlers-Danlos syndrome. Beighton P, editor. McKusick's Heritable Disorders of Connective Tissue. St. Louis: Mosby; 1992a. p. 89–251.

Beighton P. Ehlers-Danlos Syndrome. In: David TJ. Recent Advances in Paediatrics. 11th, ed. London: Churchill Livingstone; 1992b.

Beighton P. Cutis laxa. Hypertrichosis lanuginosa. Birth Defects Compendium. New York: Alan R. Liss Inc.; 1973. p. 55–559.

Beighton P, Horan FT. Surgical aspects of the Ehlers-Danlos syndrome. A survey of 100 cases. Br J Surg. 1969; 56:255–9.

Beighton P, Horan F. Orthopaedic aspects of the Ehlers Danlos syndrome. J Bone Joint Surg Br . 1969;51-B:444–453.

Beighton P, Wells RS. Ehlers-Danlos syndrome. (Two cases). Proc Roy Soc Med. 1968; 61:987–9.

Beighton P, De Paepe A, Steinmann B, Tsipouras P, Wenstrup RJ. Ehlers-Danlos syndromes: revised nosology, Villefranche, 1997. Ehlers-Danlos National Foundation (USA) and Ehlers-Danlos Support Group (UK). Am J Med Genet. 1998; 77:31–7.

Beighton P, Price A, Lord J, Dickson E. Variants of the Ehlers-Danlos syndrome. Clinical, biochemical, haematological, and chromosomal features of 100 patients. Ann Rheum Dis. 1969; 28:228–45.

Beiraghdar F, Rostami Z, Panahi Y, Einollahi B, Teimoori M. Vesicourethral reflux in pediatrics with hypermobility syndrome. Nephrourol Mon. 2013;5:924–7.

Berglund B, Nordström G, Hagberg C, Mattiasson AC. Foot pain and disability in individuals with Ehlers-Danlos syndrome (EDS): impact on daily life activities. Disabil Rehabil. 2005;27:164–9.

Berglund B, Pettersson C, Pigg M, Kristiansson P. Self-reported quality of life, anxiety and depression in individuals with Ehlers-Danlos syndrome (EDS): a questionnaire study. BMC Musculoskelet Disord. 2015;16:89.

Besteiro González JL, Suárez Fernández TV, Arboleya Rodríguez L, Muñiz J, Lemos Giráldez S, Alvarez FA. Sleep architecture in patients with fibromyalgia. Psicothema. 2011;23:368–73.

Birt L, Pfeil M, MacGregor A, Armon K, Poland F. Adherence to home physiotherapy treatment in children and young people with joint hypermobility: a qualitative report of family perspectives on acceptability and efficacy. Musculoskeletal Care. 2014;12:56–61.

Branson JA, Kozlowska K, Kaczynski KJ, Roesler TA. Managing chronic pain in a young adolescent girl with Ehlers-Danlos syndrome. Harv Rev Psychiatry. 2011;19:259–70.

Bravo JF. Síndrome de Ehlers-Danlos con especial énfasis en el síndrome de hiperlaxitud articular. Rev Med Chil. 2009;137:1488–97.

Bulbena A, Pailhez G, Bulbena-Cabré A, Mallorquí-Bagué N, Baeza-Velasco C. Joint hypermobility, anxiety and psychosomatics: two and a half decades of progress toward a new phenotype. Adv Psychosom Med. 2015;34:143–57.

Bulbena A, Baeza-Velasco C, Bulbena-Cabré A, Pailhez G, Critchley H, Chopra P, et al. Psychiatric and psychological aspects in the Ehlers-Danlos syndromes. Am J Med Genet C Semin Med Genet. 2017;175:237–45.

Burcharth J, Rosenberg J. Gastrointestinal surgery and related complications in patients with Ehlers-Danlos syndrome: a systematic review. Dig Surg. 2012;29:349–57.

Callegarini U. Clinical study on the hyperextensibility of fingers in rheumatoid children. Bull St Francis Hosp Sanat Roslyn NY. 1957;14:32.

Carter C, Sweetnam R. Familial joint laxity and recurrent dislocation of the patella. J Bone Joint Surg Br. 1958;40-B:664–7.

Carter C, Wilkinson J. Persistent joint laxity and congenital dislocation of the hip. J Bone Joint Surg Br. 1964;46:40–5.

Castori M, Camerota F, Celletti C, Danese C, Santilli V, Saraceni VM, et al. Natural history and manifestations of the hypermobility type Ehlers-Danlos syndrome: a pilot study on 21 patients. Am J Med Genet A. 2010a;152:556–64.

Castori M, Camerota F, Celletti C, Grammatico P, Padua L. Ehlers-Danlos syndrome hypermobility type and the excess of affected females: possible mechanisms and perspectives. Am J Med Genet A. 2010b;152A:2406–8.

Castori M, Sperduti I, Celletti C, Camerota F, Grammatico P. Symptom and joint mobility progression in the joint hypermobility syndrome (Ehlers–Danlos syndrome, hypermobility type). Clin Exp Rheumatol. 2011;29:998–1005.

Castori M, Morlino S, Ghibellini G, Celletti C, Camerota F, Grammatico P. Connective tissue, Ehlers-Danlos syndrome(s), and head and cervical pain. Am J Med Genet C Semin Med Genet. 2015;169C:84–96.

Castori M, Tinkle B, Levy H, Grahame R, Malfait F, Hakim A. A framework for the classification of joint hypermobility and related conditions. Am J Med Genet C Semin Med Genet. 2017;175:148–57.

Castori M, Morlino S, Celletti C, Celli M, Morrone A, Colombi M, et al. Management of pain and fatigue in the joint hypermobility syndrome (a.k.a. Ehlers-Danlos syndrome, hypermobility type): principles and proposal for a multidisciplinary approach. Am J Med Genet A. 2012;158A:2055–70.

Castori M, Morlino S, Dordoni C, Celletti C, Camerota F, Ritelli M, et al. Gynecologic and obstetric implications of the joint hypermobility syndrome (a.k.a. Ehlers–Danlos syndrome hypermobility type) in 82 Italian patients. Am J Med Genet Part A. 2012;158A:2176–82.

Castori M. Joint hypermobility syndrome (a.k.a. Ehlers-Danlos Syndrome, Hypermobility Type): an updated critique. G Ital Dermatol Venereol. 2013; 148:13–36.

Cohn P. Présentation d'un malade avec peau en caoutchouc (cutis laxa) avec des modifiations circonscrites de la peau sous formes d'elcoures brun-rouge dépressibles (IXème congrès des sociétés allemenandes de dermatologie. 1907;1907:107–415.

Connelly E, Hakim A, Davenport HS, Simmonds JV. A Study exploring the prevalence of hypermobility syndrome in a musculoskeletal triage clinic. Physiother Res Pract. 2015;36:43–53.

Czaprowski D. Generalised joint hypermobility in caucasian girls with idiopathic scoliosis: relation with age, curve size, and curve pattern. Scientific World J. 2014;2014:1–6.

Daniels AH, DePasse JM, Kamal RN. Orthopaedic surgeon burnout: Diagnosis, treatment, and prevention. J Am Acad Orthop Surg. 2016;24:213–9.

Dauvilliers Y, Touchon J. Sleep in fibromyalgia: review of clinical and polysomnographic data. Neurophysiol Clin. 2001;31:18–33.

De Paepe A, Malfait F. The Ehlers-Danlos syndrome, a disorder with many faces. Clin Genet. 2012;82:1–11.

De Coster PJ, Martens LC, De Paepe A. Oral health in prevalent types of Ehlers-Danlos syndromes. J Oral Pathol Med. 2005a;34:298–307.

De Coster PJ, Van den Berghe LI, Martens LC. Generalized joint hypermobility and temporomandibular disorders: inherited connective tissue disease as a model with maximum expression. J Orofac Pain. 2005b;19:47–57.

De Wandele I, Rombaut L, Malfait F, De Backer T, De Paepe A, Calders P. Clinical heterogeneity in patients with the hypermobility type of Ehlers-Danlos syndrome. Res Dev Disabil. 2013;34:873–81.

De Wandele I, Calders P, Peersman W, Rimbaut S, De Backer T, Malfait F, et al. Autonomic symptom burden in the hypermobility type of Ehlers-Danlos syndrome: a comparative study with two other EDS types, fibromyalgia, and healthy controls. Semin Arthritis Rheum. 2014;44:353–61.

de Kort LM, Verhulst JA, Engelbert RH, Uiterwaal CS, de Jong TP. Lower urinary tract dysfunction in children with generalized hypermobility of joints. J Urol. 2003;170:1971–4.

Delling FN, Vasan RS. Epidemiology and pathophysiology of mitral valve prolapse: new insights into disease progression, genetics, and molecular basis. Circulation. 2014;129:2158–70.

Derpapas A, Cartwright R, Upadhyaya P, Bhide AA, Digesu AG, Khullar V. Lack of association of joint hypermobility with urinary incontinence subtypes and pelvic organ prolapse. BJU Int. 2015;115:639–43.

Dickin DC, Doan JB. Postural stability in altered and unaltered sensory environments following fatiguing exercise of lower extremity joints. Scand J Med Sci Sports. 2008; 18:765–72.

Dolan AL, Mishra MB, Chambers JB, Grahame R. Clinical and echocardiographic survey of the Ehlers-Danlos syndrome. Br J Rheumatol. 1997;36:459–62.

Easton V, Bale P, Bacon H, Jerman E, Armon K, Macgregor AJ. A89: The relationship between benign joint hypermobility syndrome and developmental coordination disorders in children. Arthritis Rheum. 2014;66(Suppl 3):S124.

Eccles J, Owens A, Harrison N, Grahame R, Critchley H. Joint hypermobility and autonomic hyperactivity: an autonomic and functional neuroimaging study. Lancet. 2015;387:S40.

el-Shahaly HA, el-Sherif AK. Is the benign joint hypermobility syndrome benign? Clin Rheumatol. 1991; 10:302–7.

Ericson WB Jr, Wolman R. Orthopaedic management of the Ehlers-Danlos syndromes. Am J Med Genet C Semin Med Genet. 2017;175:188–94.

Evans AM, Rome K. A Cochrane review of the evidence for non-surgical interventions for flexible pediatric flat feet. Eur J Phys Rehabil Med. 2011;47:69–89.

Everman DB, Robin NH. Hypermobility syndrome. Pediatr Rev. 1998;19:111–7.

Falkerslev S, Baago C, Alkjær T, Remvig L, Halkjær-Kristensen J, Larsen PK, et al. Dynamic balance during gait in children and adults with Generalized Joint Hypermobility. Clin Biomech (bristol, Avon). 2013;28:318–24.

Fatoye F, Palmer S, Macmillan F, Rowe P, van der Linden M. Proprioception and muscle torque deficits in children with hypermobility syndrome. Rheumatology (oxford). 2009a;48:152–7.

Fatoye FO, Mosaku SK, Komolafe MA, Eegunranti BA, Adebayo RA, Komolafe EO, et al. Depressive symptoms and associated factors following cerebrovascular accident among Nigerians. JMH. 2009b;18:224–32.

Fikree A, Aktar R, Grahame R, Hakim AJ, Morris JK, Knowles CH, et al. Functional gastrointestinal disorders are associated with the joint hypermobility syndrome in secondary care: a case-control study. Neurogastroenterol Motil. 2015;27:569–79.

Fikree A, Chelimsky G, Collins H, Kovacic K, Aziz Q. Gastrointestinal involvement in the Ehlers-Danlos syndromes. Am J Med Genet C Semin Med Genet. 2017a;175:181–7.

Fikree A, Aziz Q, Sifrim D. Mechanisms underlying reflux symptoms and dysphagia in patients with joint hypermobility syndrome, with and without postural tachycardia syndrome. Neurogastroenterol Moil. 2017b;29: e13029.

Gazit Y, Nahir AM, Grahame R, Jacob G. Dysautonomia in the joint hypermobility syndrome. Am J Med. 2003;115:33–40.

Gazit Y, Jacob G, Grahame R. Ehlers-Danlos Syndrome-Hypermobility type: A much neglected Multisystemic Disorder. Rambam Maimonides Med J. 2016;7: e0034.

Gharbiya M, Moramarco A, Castori M, Parisi F, Celletti C, Marenco M, et al. Ocular features in joint hypermobility syndrome/ehlers-danlos syndrome hypermobility type: a clinical and in vivo confocal microscopy study. Am J Ophthalmol. 2012;154:593–600.

Goldblatt J, Wallis C, Viljoen D, Beighton P. Cutis laxa, retarded development and joint hypermobility syndrome. Dysmorph Clin Genet. 1988;1:142–4.

Grahame R. Ehlers-Danlos syndrome. S Afr Med J. 2016;106(6 Suppl 1):S45–6.

Grahame R, Beighton P. Physical properties of the skin in the Ehlers-Danlos syndrome. Ann Rheum Dis. 1969;28:246–51.

Grahame R, Beighton P. The physical properties of skin in cutis laxa. Br J Dermatol. 1971;84:326–9.

Grahame R, Bird HA, Child A. The revised (Brighton 1998) criteria for the diagnosis of joint hypermobility syndrome (BJHS). J Rheumatol. 2000;27:1777–9.

Hagberg C, Berglund B, Korpe L, Andersson-Norinder J. Ehlers-Danlos syndrome (EDS) focusing on oral symptoms: a questionnaire study. Orthod Craniofac Res. 2004;7:178–85.

Hakim AJ, Grahame R. A simple questionnaire to detect hypermobility: an adjunct to the assessment of patients with diffuse musculoskeletal pain. Int J Clin Pract. 2003;57:163–6.

Hakim AJ, Sahota A. Joint hypermobility and skin elasticity: the hereditary disorders of connective tissue. Clin Dermatol. 2006;24:521–33.

Hakim AJ, Grahame R, Norris P, Hopper C. Local anaesthetic failure in joint hypermobility syndrome. J R Soc Med. 2005;98:84–5.

Hakim A, O'Callaghan C, De Wandele I, Stiles L, Pocinki A, Rowe P. Cardiovascular autonomic dysfunction in Ehlers-Danlos syndrome-Hypermobile type. Am J Med Genet C Semin Med Genet. 2017a;175:168–74.

Hakim A, De Wandele I, O'Callaghan C, Pocinki A, Rowe P. Chronic fatigue in Ehlers-Danlos syndrome-Hypermobile type. Am J Med Genet C Semin Med Genet. 2017b;175:175–80.

Hakim AJ, Grahame R. Non-musculoskeletal symptoms in joint hypermobility syndrome. Indirect evidence for autonomic dysfunction? Rheumatology (Oxford). 2004;43:1194–5.

Hamonet C. Les douleurs dans le syndrome d'Ehlers-Danlos (à propos de 644 cas avec un test de Beighton égal ou supérieur à 4/9). J Réadaptation Médic. 2013;33:51–3.

Hamonet C, Gompel A, Mazaltarine G, Brock I, Baeza-Velasco C, Zeitoun JD, et al. Ehlers-Danlos syndrome or disease? J Syndromes. 2015;2:5.

Hamonet C, Ducret L, Layadi K, Baeza-Velasco C. Historia y Actualidad del Síndrome de EhlersDanlos-Tschernogobow. Cuad Neuropsicol. 2016;10:17–31.

Hass J, Hass R. Arthrochalasis multiplex congenita; congenital flaccidity of the joints. J Bone Joint Surg Am. 1958;40-A:663–74.

Henkel G. Strides in recognition and management of joint hypermobility syndrome [Internet]. The Rheumatologist; 2010 [cited 2017 Jul 29]. Available from: https://www.the-rheumatologist.org/article/function-despite-pain/

Hershenfeld SA, Wasim S, McNiven V, Parikh M, Majewski P, Faghfoury H, et al. Psychiatric disorders in Ehlers-Danlos syndrome are frequent, diverse and strongly associated with pain. Rheumatol Int. 2016;36:341–8.

Jacks SK, Zirwas MJ. Abnormal wound healing related to high-dose systemic corticosteroid therapy in a patient with Ehlers-Danlos syndrome benign hypermobility Type. Cutis. 2016;98:E20–3.

Jacome DE. Headache in Ehlers-Danlos syndrome. Cephalalgia. 1999;19:791–6.

Jansson A, Saartok T, Werner S, Renstrom P. General joint laxity in 1845 Swedish school children of different ages: age- and gender-specific distributions. Acta Paediatr. 2004;93:1202–6.

Kemp S, Roberts I, Gamble C, Wilkinson S, Davidson JE, Baildam EM, et al. A randomized comparative trial of generalized vs targeted physiotherapy in the management of childhood hypermobility. Rheumatology (oxford). 2010;49:315–25.

Kerr A, Macmillan CE, Uttley WS, Luqmani RA. Physiotherapy for children with hypermobility syndrome. Physiotherapy. 2000;86:313–7.

Kirby A, Davies R. Developmental Coordination disorder and joint hypermobility syndrome–overlapping disorders? Implications for research and clinical practice. Child Care Health Dev. 2007;33:513–9.

Kirby A, Davies R, Bryant A. Hypermobility syndrome and developmental coordination disorder: similarities and features. Int J Ther Rehabil. 2005;12:431–7.

Kirk JA, Ansell BM, Bywaters EG. The hypermobility syndrome. Musculoskeletal complaints associated with generalized joint hypermobility. Ann Rheum Dis. 1967; 26:419–25.

Korterink JJ, Ockeloen L, Benninga MA, Tabbers MM, Hilbink M, Deckers-Kocken JM. Probiotics for childhood functional gastrointestinal disorders: a systematic review and meta-analysis. Acta Paediatr. 2014;103:365–72.

Kozanoglu E, Coskun Benlidayi I, Eker Akilli R, Tasal A. Is there any link between joint hypermobility and mitral valve prolapse in patients with fibromyalgia syndrome? Clin Rheumatol. 2016;35:1041–4.

Landry BW, Fischer PR, Driscoll SW, Koch KM, Harbeck-Weber C, Mack KJ, et al. Managing chronic pain in children and adolescents: a clinical review. PMR. 2015;7(11 Suppl):S295-315.

Lamari et al. No Prelo 2022.

Levine SA. Clinical heart disease. 5th ed. Philadelphia: Saunders; 1958. p. 12.

Mack KJ. Management of chronic daily headache in children. Expert Rev Neurother. 2010;10:1479–86.

Maeland S, Assmus J, Berglund B. Subjective health complaints in individuals with Ehlers Danlos syndrome: a questionnaire study. Int J Nurs Stud. 2011;48:720–4.

Malfait F, Syx D, Vlummens P, Symoens S, Nampoothiri S, Hermanns-Lê T, et al. Musculocontractural Ehlers-Danlos Syndrome (former EDS type VIB) and adducted thumb clubfoot syndrome (ATCS) represent a single clinical entity caused by mutations in the dermatan-4-sulfotransferase 1 encoding CHST14 gene. Hum Mutat. 2010;31:1233–9.

Malfait F, Francomano C, Byers P, Belmont J, Berglund B, Black J, et al. The 2017 international classification of the Ehlers-Danlos syndromes. Am J Med Genet C Semin Med Genet. 2017;175:8–26.

Malfait F, Castori M, Francomano CA, Giunta C, Kosho T, Byers PH. As síndromes de Ehlers-Danlos. Primers Nat Rev Dis. 2020;6(1):64.

Mallik AK, Ferrell WR, McDonald AG, Sturrock RD. Impaired proprioceptive acuity at the proximal interphalangeal joint in patients with the hypermobility syndrome. Br J Rheumatol. 1994;33:631–7.

Marino LHC, Lamari N, Marino NW Jr. Hipermobilidade articular nos joelhos da criança. Arq Ciênc Saúde. 2004;11:124–7.

Massie WK, Howorth MB. Congenital dislocation of the hip. Part III. Pathogenesis. J Bone Joint Surg Am. 1951;33A:190–8.

Mathias CJ, Low DA, Iodice V, Owens AP, Kirbis M, Grahame R. Postural tachycardia syndrome–current experience and concepts. Nat Rev Neurol. 2011;8:22–34.

McDonnell NB, Gorman BL, Mandel KW, Schurman SH, Assanah-Carroll A, Mayer SA, et al. Echocardiographic findings in classical and hypermobile Ehlers-Danlos syndromes. Am J Med Genet A. 2006;140:129–36.

McIntosh LJ, Mallett VT, Frahm JD, Richardson DA, Evans MI. Gynecologic disorders in women with Ehlers-Danlos syndrome. J Soc Gynecol Investig. 1995;2:559–64.

Mckusick VA. Heritable disorders of connective tissue: Iv the Ehlers-Danlos syndrome. J Chronic Dis. 1956;3:2–24.

McKusick VA. Heritable disorders of connective tissue. 3rd ed. St. Louis: Mosby; 1966. p. 47.

Mckusick VA. Heritable disorders of connective tissue. St Louis: Mosby Company; 1972.

Milhorat TH, Bolognese PA, Nishikawa M, McDonnell NB, Francomano CA. Syndrome of occipitoatlantoaxial hypermobility, cranial settling, and chiari malformation type I in patients with hereditary disorders of connective tissue. J Neurosurg Spine. 2007;7:601–9.

Mintz-Itkin R, Lerman-Sagie T, Zuk L, Itkin-Webman T, Davidovitch M. Does physical therapy improve outcome in infants with joint hypermobility and benign hypotonia? J Child Neurol. 2009;24:714–9.

Mulvey MR, Macfarlane GJ, Beasley M, Symmons DP, Lovell K, Keeley P, et al. Modest association of joint hypermobility with disabling and limiting musculoskeletal pain: results from a large-scale general population-based survey. Arthritis Care Res (hoboken). 2013;65:1325–33.

Murray B, Yashar BM, Uhlmann WR, Clauw DJ, Petty EM. Ehlers-Danlos syndrome, hypermobility type: a characterization of the patients' lived experience. Am J Med Genet A. 2013;161A:2981–8.

Myer GD, Ford KR, Paterno MV, Nick TG, Hewett TE. The effects of generalized joint laxity on risk of anterior cruciate ligament injury in young female athletes. Am J Sports Med. 2008;36:1073–80.

Neilson D, Martin VT. Joint hypermobility and headache: understanding the glue that binds the two together—Part 1. Headache. 2014;54:1393–402.

Nelson JA, Fischer J, Chung CC, Wink J, Wes A, Serletti JM, et al. Readmission following ventral hernia repair: a model derived from the ACS-NSQIP datasets. Hernia. 2015;19:125–33.

Nosouhian S, Haghighat A, Mohammadi I, Shadmehr E, Davoudi A, Badrian H. Temporomandibular joint hypermobility manifestation based on clinical observations. J Intl Oral Health. 2015;7:1–4.

Ofluoglu D, Gunduz OH, Kul-Panza E, Guven Z. Hypermobility in women with fibromyalgia syndrome. Clin Rheuamtol. 2006;25:291–3.

Pacey V, Tofts L, Adams RD, Munns CF, Nicholson LL. Exercise in children with joint hypermobility syndrome and knee pain: a randomised controlled trial comparing exercise into hypermobile versus neutral knee extension. Pediatr Rheumatol Online J. 2013;11:30.

Pacey V, Tofts L, Adams RD, Munns CF, Nicholson LL. Quality of life prediction in children with joint hypermobility syndrome. J Paediatr Child Health. 2015;51:689–95.

Parapia LA, Jackson C. Ehlers-Danlos syndrome - a historical review. Br J Haematol. 2008;141:32–5.

Rahman N, Dunstan M, Teare MD, Hanks S, Douglas J, Coleman K, et al. Ehlers-Danlos syndrome with severe early-onset periodontal disease (EDS-VIII) is a distinct, heterogeneous disorder with one predisposition gene at chromosome 12p13. Am J Hum Genet. 2003;73:198–204.

Ramesh R, Von Arx O, Azzopardi T, Schranz PJ. The risk of anterior cruciate ligament rupture with generalised joint laxity. J Bone Joint Surg Br. 2005;87:800–3.

Rigoldi C, Galli M, Cimolin V, Camerota F, Celletti C, Tenore N, et al. Gait strategy in patients with Ehlers-Danlos syndrome hypermobility type and Down syndrome. Res Dev Disabil. 2012;33:437–42.

Rombaut L, De Paepe A, Malfait F, Cools A, Calders P. Joint position sense and vibratory perception sense in patients with Ehlers-Danlos syndrome type III (hypermobility type). Clin Rheumatol. 2010a;29:289–95.

Rombaut L, Malfait F, Cools A, De Paepe A, Calders P. Musculoskeletal complaints, physical activity and health-related quality of life among patients with the Ehlers-Danlos syndrome hypermobility type. Disabil Rehabil. 2010b;32:1339–45.

Rombaut L, Malfait F, De Paepe A, Rimbaut S, Verbruggen G, De Wandele I, et al. Impairment and impact of pain in female patients with Ehlers-Danlos syndrome: a comparative study with fibromyalgia and rheumatoid arthritis. Arthritis Rheum. 2011a;63:1979–87.

Rombaut L, Malfait F, De Wandele I, Cools A, Thijs Y, De Paepe A, et al. Medication, surgery, and physiotherapy among patients with the hypermobility type of Ehlers-Danlos syndrome. Arch Phys Med Rehabil. 2011b;92:1106–12.

Rombaut L, Malfait F, De Wandele I, Mahieu N, Thijs Y, Segers P, et al. Muscle-tendon tissue properties in the hypermobility type of Ehlers-Danlos syndrome. Arthritis Care Res (hoboken). 2012a;64:766–72.

Rombaut L, Malfait F, De Wandele I, Taes Y, Thijs Y, De Paepe A, et al. Muscle mass, muscle strength, functional performance, and physical impairment in women with the hypermobility type of Ehlers-Danlos syndrome. Arthritis Care Res (hoboken). 2012b;64:1584–92.

Ronchese F. Dermatorrhexis, with dermatochalasis and arthrochalasis (the so-called Ehlers-Danlos syndrome). Am J Dis Child. 1936;51:1403.

Rose KA, Morgan IG, Ip J, Kifley A, Huynh S, Smith W, et al. Outdoor activity reduces the prevalence of myopia in children. Ophthalmology. 2008;115:1279–85.

Ross A, Hauser MD, Phillips HJ. Treatment of Joint Hypermobility Syndrome, including Ehlers-Danlos Syndrome, with Hackett-Hemwall Prolotherapy. J Prolotherapy. 2011;3:612–29.

Rowe P, Barron D, Calkins H, Maumenee I, Tong P, Geraghty M. Orthostatic intolerance and chronic fatigue syndrome associated with Ehlers-Danlos syndrome. J Pediatr. 1999;135:494–9.

Rozen TD, Roth JM, Denenberg N. Cervical spine joint hypermobility: a possible predisposing factor for new daily persistent headache. Cephalalgia. 2006;26:1182–5.

Scheper MC, de Vries JE, de Vos R, Verbunt J, Nollet F, Engelbert RH. Generalized joint hypermobility in professional dancers: a sign of talent or vulnerability? Rheumatology (oxford). 2013;52:651–8.

Scheper MC, Juul-Kristensen B, Rombaut L, Rameckers EA, Verbunt J, Engelbert RH. Disability in adolescents and adults diagnosed with hypermobility-related disorders: a meta-analysis. Arch Phys Med Rehabil. 2016;97:2174–87.

Schubert-Hjalmarsson E, Ohman A, Kyllerman M, Beckung E. Pain, balance, activity, and participation in children with hypermobility syndrome. Pediatr Phys Ther. 2012;24:339–44.

Shirley ED, Demaio M, Bodurtha J. Ehlers-danlos syndrome in orthopaedics: etiology, diagnosis, and treatment implications. Sports Health. 2012;4:394–403.

Simmonds JV, Keer RJ. Hypermobility and the hypermobility syndrome. Man Ther. 2007;12:298–309.

Simpson MR. Benign joint hypermobility syndrome: evaluation, diagnosis, and management. J Am Osteopath Assoc. 2006;106:531–6.

Sinibaldi L, Ursini G, Castori M. Psychopathological manifestations of joint hypermobility and joint hypermobility syndrome/ Ehlers-Danlos syndrome, hypermobility type: The link between connective tissue and psychological distress revised. Am J Med Genet C Semin Med Genet. 2015;169C:97–106.

Sipilä K, Suominen AL, Alanen P, Heliövaara M, Tiittanen P, Könönen M. Association of clinical findings of temporomandibular disorders (TMD) with self-reported musculoskeletal pains. Eur J Pain. 2011;15:1061–7.

Sparto PJ, Parnianpour M, Reinsel TE, Simon S. The effect of fatigue on multijoint kinematics, coordination, and postural stability during a repetitive lifting test. J Orthopaedic Sport Phys Therap. 1997;25:3–12.

Stanitski DF, Nadjarian R, Stanitski CL, Bawle E, Tsipouras P. Orthopaedic manifestations of Ehlers-Danlos syndrome. Clin Orthop. 2000;376:213–21.

Stern CM, Pepin MJ, Stoler JM, Kramer DE, Spencer SA, Stein CJ. Musculoskeletal conditions in a pediatric population with Ehlers-Danlos syndrome. J Pediatr. 2016;181:261–6.

Sutro CJ. Hypermobility of bones due to "overlengthened" capsular and ligamentous tissues; a cause for recurrent intra-articular effusions. Surgery. 1947;21:67.

Tapley E, Beighton P. Calcification of breast tissue in the Ehlers-Danlos syndrome. Breast J. 2009;15:537–9.

Ting TV, Hashkes PJ, Schikler K, Desai AM, Spalding S, Kashikar-Zuck S. The role of benign joint hypermobility in the pain experience in juvenile fibromyalgia: an observational study. Pediatr Rheumatol Online J. 2012;10:16.

Tinkle BT. Joint hypermobility handbook- a guide for the issues and management of Ehlers-Danlos syndrome hypermobility type and the hypermobility syndrome. Niles (IL): Left Paw Press; 2010.

Tinkle B, Castori M, Berglund B, Cohen H, Grahame R, Kazkaz H, et al. Hypermobile Ehlers-Danlos syndrome (a.k.a. Ehlers-Danlos syndrome Type III and Ehlers-Danlos syndrome hypermobility type): clinical description and natural history. Am J Med Genet C Semin Med Genet. 2017; 175:48–69.

Tobias N. Danlos syndrome associated with congenital lipomatosis. Arch Derm Syphilol. 1934;30:540.

Tobias JH, Deere K, Palmer S, Clark EM, Clinch J. Joint hypermobility is a risk factor for musculoskeletal pain during adolescence: findings of a prospective cohort study. Arthritis Rheum. 2013;65:1107–15.

Viljoen D, Goldblatt J, Thompson D, Beighton P. Ehlers-Danlos syndrome: yet another type? Clin Genet. 1987;32:196–201.

Voermans NC, Knoop H, Bleijenberg G, van Engelen BG. Pain in ehlers-danlos syndrome is common, severe, and associated with functional impairment. J Pain Symptom Manage. 2010;40:370–8.

Voermans NC, Knoop H, Bleijenberg G, van Engelen BG. Fatigue is associated with muscle weakness in Ehlers-Danlos syndrome: an explorative study. Physiotherapy. 2011;97:170–4.

Volkov N, Nisenblat V, Ohel G, Gonen R. Ehlers-Danlos syndrome: insights on obstetric aspects. Obstet Gynecol Surv. 2007;62:51–7.

Walker BA, Beighton P, Lamont MJ. The Marfanoid hypermobility syndrome. Ann Int Med. 1969;71:349–52.

Weber FP. The Ehlers-Danlos syndrome. Br J Dermatol Syph. 1936;48:609.

Wijnhoven HA, de Vet HC, Picavet HS. Explaining sex differences in chronic musculoskeletal pain in a general population. Pain. 2006;124:158–66.

Zarate N, Farmer AD, Grahame R, Mohammed SD, Knowles CH, Scott SM, et al. Unexplained gastrointestinal symptoms and joint hypermobility: is connective tissue the missing link? Neurogastroenterol Motil. 2010;22:252-e78.

Zweers MC, Bristow J, Steijlen PM, Dean WB, Hamel BC, Otero M, et al. of TNXB is associated with hypermobility type of Ehlers-Danlos syndrome. Am J Hum Genet. 2003;73:214–7.

8

Joint Hypermobility Syndrome and Hypermobility Spectrum Disorders

Hypermobility Spectrum Disorders as Updated Diagnosis of the Ehlers-Danlos Syndrome, Hypermobility Type, and Joint Hypermobility Syndrome

As suggested by Castori et al. (2017) the hypermobility spectrum disorders (Hsds) are a group of clinical conditions related to joint hypermobility (JH) that are descriptive and of diagnostic exclusion. They are used mainly as alternative labels for patients with symptomatic JH who do not meet the criteria of a variant of Ehlers-Danlos syndrome (EDS). The hypermobile form (hEDS) is defined in terms of severity, musculoskeletal involvement pattern, and/or due to the absence of other necessary criteria, as reported in the new nosology for Ehlers-Danlos syndromes (EDS). The term "HSDs" also refers to a broad

N. Lamari and P. Beighton, *Hypermobility in Medical Practice*,
In Clinical Practice, https://doi.org/10.1007/978-3-031-34914-0_8

gamut of musculoskeletal manifestations that may be considered "secondary" to the underlying JH.

The categorization of the spectrum of disorders related to JH is most often congenital, possibly an inherited trait with phenotypic domains of HSDs generally limited to the musculoskeletal system. This includes the presence of one or more articular and extra-articular manifestations that are secondary to JH. The molecular basis remains unknown and the aetiopathogenesis of these manifestations is complex due to a variety of acquired factors.

The term "HSDs" may become the updated diagnosis for all individuals who meet the previous criteria for the hypermobile type of EDS or joint hypermobility syndrome (JHS) but do not correspond to the proposed criteria for hEDS. However, the term HSDs is used to identify discrete subtypes that fill the gap between asymptomatic JH and hEDS. These HSDs warrant consideration including the possibility of the clinical evolution and the transition to another diagnosis (such as, hEDS).

Proposed Classification for the Spectrum of Disorders Related to Joint Hypermobility

A group of four different HSDs have been identified as components of the joint hypermobility spectrum:

1. Generalized HSD (G-HSD): Generalized JH is evaluated using the Beighton score plus one or more secondary musculoskeletal manifestations. This category includes those persons who do not meet the diagnostic criteria for hEDS.

2. Peripheral HSD (P-HSD): JH is limited to the hands and feet plus one or more secondary musculoskeletal manifestations.
3. Localized HSD (L-HSD): JH is identified in single joints or a group of joints plus one or more secondary musculoskeletal manifestations.
4. Historical HSD (HSD-H): Self-reported (historical) generalized JH using a five-point questionnaire (Hakim and Grahame 2003) when the Beighton score (Beighton et al. 1973) is negative, plus one or more secondary musculoskeletal manifestations with the exclusion of alternative diagnoses of G-HSD, P-HSD and L-HSD, as well as other articular and rheumatological conditions.

Musculoskeletal Manifestations Secondary to Joint Hypermobility

Musculoskeletal patterns related to JH include joint manifestations, which are highly variable and strongly related to modifying factors, such as gender (Malfait et al. 2006; Flowers et al. 2018) mechanical forces (Castori et al. 2017; Ericson and Wolman 2017) personal habits (O'Sullivan et al. 2017) work activities (Lewańska et al. 2016; Gyer et al. 2018) accidents (Schwarz et al. 1993; Rombaut et al. 2011) and sports activities (Nathan et al. 2018). The manifestations are causally independent of JH and may emerge at different ages (Castori and Colombi 2015; Morlino et al. 2017). It follows that, such manifestations are not due to the underlying cause of JH and have secondary effects mediated by JH and other factors (Castori et al. 2017; Ericson and Wolman 2017).

Secondary manifestations of JH include pain, degenerative joint and bone disease. Neurodevelopment features (Ghibellini et al. 2015) muscle weakness, proprioceptive deficit (Ericson and Wolman 2017) and trauma (Groh and Herrera 2009; Tobias et al. 2013; Tinkle et al. 2017). Other musculoskeletal features may occur as the result of the JH trait. Among these are macro-trauma and microtrauma (Ericson and Wolman 2017). Macro-trauma includes luxation/subluxation (Tobias et al. 2013; Gazit et al. 2016) and soft tissue damage (ligaments, tendons, and muscles) (Henkel and Strides 2010). This type of trauma can cause acute pain and the loss of joint function (Ericson and Wolman 2017). Microtraumas are very small injuries with a cumulative effect perceived over time that can lead to recurrent or persistent pain and possibly premature joint degeneration which evolves into osteoarthritis (Coster et al. 2005; Groh and Herrera 2009; Tinkle et al. 2017).

Other Joint and Musculoskeletal Characteristics Associated with Generalized Joint Hypermobility

Other musculoskeletal manifestations associated with generalized JH are often the signs and symptoms of minor physical traits that may be the result of interactions between "softer" musculoskeletal tissues and mechanical forces during growth. These include flat feet, misaligned bones, mild to moderate scoliosis, mild to moderate kyphosis of the upper part of the spine, and mild to moderate lordosis of the lower spine (Jasiewicz et al. 2010). There may be an indirect association with a mild reduction in bone mass, which may partially be explained by impaired proprioception and muscle weakness. It is also necessary to consider reduction in physical activity beginning in childhood, as affected individuals avoid recreational and sports activities, and often remain seated or lying down in functionally and esthetically inappropriate positions, with a tendency toward social isolation.

Extra-Articular Manifestations as Comorbidities Related to Joint Hypermobility

Manifestations in other organs and tissues may occur in affected persons, particularly in the form of comorbidities related to JH, which are extra-articular manifestations (Veit-Rubin et al. 2016; Bulbena et al. 2017; Fikree et al. 2017); Hakim et al. 2017. In these conditions the clinical manifestations do not meet the criteria for any of the different types of EDS and are not the direct result of the abnormal mechanics of JH. However, these factors exert a considerable negative impact on the quality of life of affected persons and their families (Sinibaldi et al. 2015).

There is an association between generalized JH and specific extra-articular conditions. The most frequent of which are anxiety disorders (Henkel and Strides in, 2010; Sinibaldi et al. 2015; Bulbena et al. 2017) orthostatic tachycardia (Mathias et al. 2011; Lamari et al. 2020) functional gastrointestinal disorders (Zarate et al. 2010; Fikree et al. 2017) pelvic disorders and bladder dysfunction (Kort et al. 2003; Tinkle 2010; Veit-Rubin et al. 2016). These associations are often encountered in clinical practice and are clinically relevant, as they are commonly found in conditions involving JH, particularly hEDS. They exert considerable impact on the quality of life and in the management of affected individuals (Castori et al. 2017). Such manifestations can also occur as comorbidities related to JH in patients with HSDs.

References

Beighton P, Solomon L, Soskolne CL. Articular mobility in an African population. Ann Rheum Dis. 1973;32(5):413–8. https://doi.org/10.1136/ard.32.5.413.

Bulbena A, Baeza-Velasco C, Bulbena-Cabré A, Pailhez G, Critchley H, Chopra P, et al. Psychiatric and psychological aspects in the Ehlers-Danlos syndromes. Am J Med Genet C Semin Med Genet. 2017;175(1):237–45. https://doi.org/10.1002/ajmg.c.31544.

Castori M, Colombi M. Generalized joint hypermobility, joint hypermobility syndrome and Ehlers-Danlos syndrome, hypermobility type. Am J Med Genet C Semin Med Genet. 2015;169C(1):1–5. https://doi.org/10.1002/ajmg.c.31432.

Castori M, Tinkle B, Levy H, Grahame R, Malfait F, Hakim A. A framework for the classification of joint hypermobility and related conditions. Am J Med Genet C Semin Med Genet. 2017;175(1):148–57. https://doi.org/10.1002/ajmg.c.31539.

De Coster PJ, Van den Berghe LI, Martens LC. Generalized joint hypermobility and temporomandibular disorders: inherited connective tissue disease as a model with maximum expression. J Orofac Pain. 2005;19(1):47–57.

De Kort LM, Verhulst JA, Engelbert RH, Uiterwaal CS, De Jong TP. Lower urinary tract dysfunction in children with generalized hypermobility of joints. J Urol. 2003;170(5):1971–4. https://doi.org/10.1097/01.ju.0000091643.35118.d3.

Ericson WB Jr, Wolman R. Orthopaedic management of the Ehlers-Danlos syndromes. Am J Med Genet C Semin Med Genet. 2017;175(1):188–94. https://doi.org/10.1002/ajmg.c.31551.

Fikree A, Aziz Q, Sifrim D. Mechanisms underlying reflux symptoms and dysphagia in patients with joint hypermobility syndrome, with and without postural tachycardia syndrome. Neurogastroenterol Motil. 2017;29(6). https://doi.org/10.1111/nmo.13029.

Flowers PPE, Cleveland RJ, Schwartz TA, Schwartz TA, Nelson AE, Kraus VB, et al. Association between general joint hypermobility and knee, hip, and lumbar spine osteoarthritis by race: a cross-sectional study. Arthritis Res Ther. 2018;20(1):76. https://doi.org/10.1186/s13075-018-1570-7.

Gazit Y, Jacob G, Grahame R. Ehlers-Danlos syndrome-hypermobility type: a much neglected multisystemic disorder. Rambam Maimonides Med J. 2016;7(4): e0034. https://doi.org/10.5041/RMMJ.10261.

Ghibellini G, Brancati F, Castori M. Neurodevelopmental attributes of joint hypermobility syndrome/Ehlers-Danlos syndrome, hypermobility type: update and perspectives. Am J Med Genet C Semin Med Genet. 2015;169C(1):107–16. https://doi.org/10.1002/ajmg.c.31424.

Groh MM, Herrera J. A comprehensive review of hip labral tears. Curr Rev Musculoskelet Med. 2009;2(2):105–17. https://doi.org/10.1007/s12178-009-9052-9.

Gyer G, Michael J, Inklebarger J. Occupational hand injuries: a current review of the prevalence and proposed prevention strategies for physical therapists and similar healthcare professionals. J Integr Med. 2018;16(2):84–9. https://doi.org/10.1016/j.joim.2018.02.003.

Hakim AJ, Grahame R. A simple questionnaire to detect hypermobility: an adjunct to the assessment of patients with diffuse musculoskeletal pain. Int J Clin Pract. 2003;57(3):163–6.

Hakim A, O'Callaghan C, De Wandele I, Stiles L, Pocinki A, Rowe P. Cardiovascular autonomic dysfunction in Ehlers-Danlos Syndrome-Hypermobile type. Am J Med Genet C Semin Med Genet. 2017;175(1):168–74. https://doi.org/10.1002/ajmg.c.31543.

Henkel G. Strides in recognition and management of joint hypermobility syndrome. 2010. Disponível em: http://www.the-rheumatologist.org/article/function-despite-pain/?singlepage=1&theme=print-friendly. Acesso em : 29 July 2017.

Jasiewicz B, Potaczek T, Tesiorowski M, Lokas K. Spine deformities in patients with Ehlers-Danlos syndrome, type IV - late results of surgical treatment. Scoliosis. 2010;5:26. https://doi.org/10.1186/1748-7161-5-26.

Lamari N, Lamari M, Medeiros MP, Pavarino EC. Signs and symptoms in children and adolescents with joint hypermobility: an observational, quantitative cross-sectional study. Rev Chil Rheumatol. 2020;36(2):42–53.

Lewańska M, Grzegorzewski A, Walusiak-Skorupa J. Bilateral hypermobility of ulnar nerves at the elbow joint with unilateral left ulnar neuropathy in a computer user: a case study. Int J Occup Med Environ Health. 2016;29(3):517–22. https://doi.org/10.13075/ijomeh.1896.00398.

Malfait F, Hakim AJ, De Paepe A, Grahame R. The genetic basis of the joint hypermobility syndromes. Rheumatology (Oxford). 2006;45(5):502–7. https://doi.org/10.1093/rheumatology/kei268.

Mathias CJ, Low DA, Iodice V, Owens AP, Kirbis M, Grahame R. Postural tachycardia syndrome–current experience and concepts. Nat Rev Neurol. 2011;8(1):22–34. https://doi.org/10.1038/nrneurol.2011.187.

Morlino S, Dordoni C, Sperduti I, Venturini M, Celletti C, Camerota F, et al. Refining patterns of joint hypermobility, habitus, and orthopedic traits in joint hypermobility syndrome and Ehlers-Danlos syndrome, hypermobility type. Am J Med Genet A. 2017;173(4):914–29. https://doi.org/10.1002/ajmg.a.38106.

Nathan JA, Davies K, Swaine I. Hypermobility and sports injury. BMJ Open Sport Exerc Med. 2018;4(1): e000366. https://doi.org/10.1136/bmjsem-2018-000366.

O'Sullivan P, Smith A, Beales D, Straker L. Understanding adolescent low back pain from a multidimensional perspective: implications for management. J Orthop Sports Phys Ther. 2017;47(10):741–51. https://doi.org/10.2519/jospt.2017.7376.

Rombaut L, Malfait F, De Wandele I, Thijs Y, Palmans T, De Paepe A, et al. Balance, gait, falls, and fear of falling in women with the hypermobility type of Ehlers-Danlos syndrome. Arthritis Care Res (hoboken). 2011;63(10):1432–9. https://doi.org/10.1002/acr.20557.

Schwarz N, Ohner T, Schwarz AF, Gerschpacher M, Meznik A. Injuries of the cervical spine in children and adolescents]. Unfallchirurg. 1993;96(5):235–41. German.

Sinibaldi L, Ursini G, Castori M. Psychopathological manifestations of joint hypermobility and joint hypermobility syndrome/ Ehlers-Danlos syndrome, hypermobility type: the link between connective tissue and psychological distress revised. Am J Med Genet C Semin Med Genet. 2015;169C(1):97–106. https://doi.org/10.1002/ajmg.c.31430.

Tinkle BT. Joint Hypermobility Handbook-A Guide for the Issues and Management of Ehlers-Danlos Syndrome Hypermobility Type and the Hypermobility Syndrome. Niles (IL): Left Paw Press; 2010.

Tinkle B, Castori M, Berglund B, Cohen H, Grahame R, Kazkaz H, et al. Hypermobile Ehlers-Danlos syndrome (a.k.a. Ehlers-Danlos syndrome type III and Ehlers-Danlos syndrome hypermobility type): clinical description and natural history. Am J Med Genet C Semin Med Genet. 2017;175(1):48–69. https://doi.org/10.1002/ajmg.c.31538.

Tobias JH, Deere K, Palmer S, Clark EM, Clinch J. Joint hypermobility is a risk factor for musculoskeletal pain during adolescence: findings of a prospective cohort study. Arthritis Rheum. 2013;65(4):1107–15. https://doi.org/10.1002/art.37836.

Veit-Rubin N, Cartwright R, Singh AU, Digesu GA, Fernando R, Khullar V. Association between joint hypermobility and pelvic organ prolapse in women: a systematic review and meta-analysis. Int Urogynecol J. 2016;27(10):1469–78. https://doi.org/10.1007/s00192-015-2896-1.

Zarate N, Farmer AD, Grahame R, Mohammed SD, Knowles CH, Scott SM, et al. Unexplained gastrointestinal symptoms and joint hypermobility: is connective tissue the missing link? Neurogastroenterol Motil. 2010;22(3):252-e78. https://doi.org/10.1111/j.1365-2982.2009.01421.x.

9

Joint Hypermobility in Different Periods of Life; An Overview

Musculoskeletal Manifestations of Preclinical and Clinical Stages of Joint Hypermobility

In the first year of life, the locomotor system of children with JH can exhibit characteristics with implications for neuropsychomotor development (Engelbert et al. 2003; Scheper et al. 2013; Lamari et al. 2020). For this reason, it is necessary to investigate the cause of ill health in affected families.

A proportion of affected children may experience serious musculoskeletal manifestations, affecting the facial profile, oral health, the spinal column, and the limbs (Mitakides and Tinkle 2017; Goode et al. 2019; Gullo et al. 2019; Russek et al. 2019). Extra-skeletal manifestations such as gastrointestinal disorders may also be associated. Nevertheless, affected children are likely to develop

N. Lamari and P. Beighton, *Hypermobility in Medical Practice*, In Clinical Practice, https://doi.org/10.1007/978-3-031-34914-0_9

avoidable physical disabilities, having exhibited minor signs since birth (Fig. 9.1). These manifestations may include poor physical performance compared with other children, leading to exclusion from recreative, sport, and social activities.

The physical signs of hypermobility include motor and cognitive deficits, benign motor delay (Mintz-Itkin et al. 2009) frequent falls (Rombaut et al. 2011) attention deficit (Baeza-Velasco et al. 2018) apathy (El-Metwally et al. 2007; Mallorquí-Bagué et al. 2014) hyperactivity (Glans et al. 2017; Baeza-Velasco et al. 2018) fatigue (Wandele et al. 2016; Russek et al. 2019) leg pain (Chopra et al. 2017; Peterson et al. 2018; Lamari et al. 2020) and abdominal region pain (Metwally et al. 2007; Mintz-Itkin et al. 2009; Rombaut et al. 2011; El-Mallorquí-Bagué et al. 2014; Castori et al. 2015; Wandele et al. 2016; Chopra et al. 2017; Glans et al. 2017; Mitakides and Tinkle 2017; Baeza-Velasco et al. 2018; Peterson et al. 2018; Goode et al. 2019; Gullo et al. 2019; Russek et al. 2019; Lamari et al. 2020). There may also be a history of bullying by family, friends, and schoolmates. These issues can change the course of the lives of affected individuals and their families due to a lack of awareness on the underlying problem.

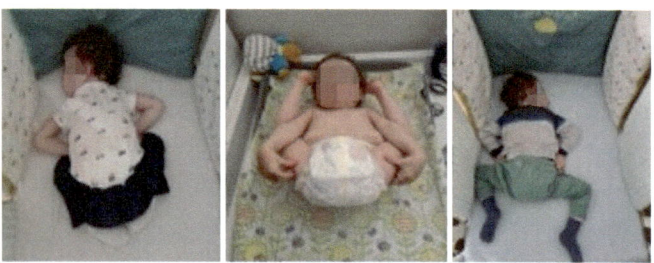

Fig. 9.1 Atypical ability of a hypermobile child

In most newborns with JH, insufficient robustness in the structure of tissues can be identified through inspection, palpation, and special physical-clinical tests. These manifestations remain throughout the preschool and school phases and are observed by educators and often by the parents themselves, but sometimes misunderstood (Lamari et al. 2020, 2022).

In adolescence, physical signs progress quickly and become defined by adulthood (Seçkin et al. 2005; Morris et al. 2017) In this phase, clothing covers the body structures of affected adolescents and sometimes neither parents nor teachers identify the problems. However, it is a rapid period with no reversal and it can change the course of these individual's lives, both physically and emotionally, causing long term suffering (Godwin et al. 2018).

Children and adolescents with signs and symptoms of JH pose a challenge to therapists in terms of effective management. In the multidisciplinary team, physiotherapists are recognized for their central role in the management of individuals with disorders related to hypermobility due to the implications with regards to body mechanics (Simmonds and Keer 2007; Grahame and Hakim 2008; Fatoye et al. 2009; Palmer et al. 2014; Scheper et al. 2016).

Young adults suffer the consequences of these deformities together with potentiation of other symptoms associated with JH (Bravo 2009; Castori and Hakim 2017). They often use medications that do little or nothing to solve the underlying problem. During this period, the implications of the lack of early intervention become evident (Lamari et al. 2022).

Elderly people suffer the consequences of progressive deformities of the spine and limbs (Goode et al. 2019; Gullo et al. 2019) the majority of which may have begun in childhood or adolescence. There is the possibility of becoming physically disabled. Nevertheless, it is relevant that a person with JH does not necessarily develop deformities.

The majority of elderly individuals with undiagnosed JH have joint deformities that impose limitations on the majority of activities of daily living. Instrumental, recreational, sport, and occupational pursuits may also be compromised. For these reasons the health of individuals with JH depends on promotion and prevention actions in childhood and adolescence (Lamari et al. 2022).

Implications of Inadequate Postural Habits in Individuals with Joint Hypermobility in Different Periods of Life

Individuals with JH are more vulnerable to microtraumas (Jasiewicz et al. 2010; Nourissat et al. 2018; Tibbo et al. 2019;) and macrotraumas (Wolf et al. 2011) and eventually adopt inadequate postural habits (Vařeková et al. 2011; Rietveld 2013; Juul-Kristensen et al. 2016). This process results in the insufficient support of the physiological function of the locomotor apparatus (Lamari et al. 2022). It is relevant that tissues may undergo degenerative processes (Yao et al. 2013) with silent, insidious signs and symptoms (Sperotto et al. 2014).

The postural pattern of individuals with JH results from the increased range of motion of certain joints, leading to instinctive postural habits in the sitting and lying positions (Fig. 9.2). Therefore, it compromises specific body regions (e.g., the hands) that are inadequate for the proper development and maturity of tissues and bone structures, more specifically the spine and lower limbs (Sperotto et al. 2014).

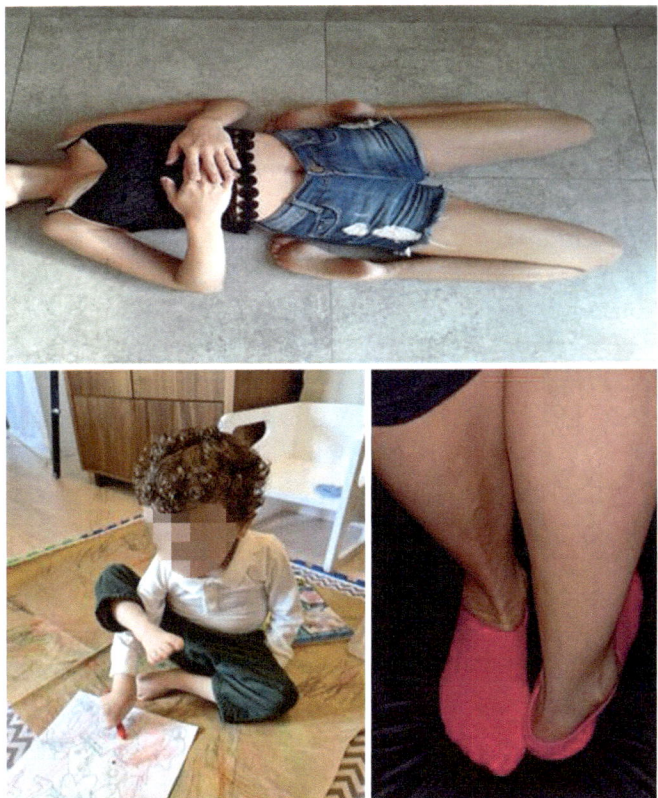

Fig. 9.2 Habits of inappropriate postures in people with JH

This pattern of joint involvement results in several well-defined physical factors and implications regarding other features which result from inadequate postures (Russek et al. 2019). These inadequacies include unsuitable footwear (Bálint et al. 2003) and seats (Gal-Nadasan et al. 2017) which further enhance the deviations of the vertebral axis (e.g., scoliosis and straightening of the vertebral axis curves) (Wong et al. 2017) hip joint incongruence, injury of the acetabular labrum (Clavert 2015) and deformities of the knees (genu recurvatum) (Marino et al. 2004; Junge et al. 2015) ankles, toes (valgus hallux and spaced toes) (Lui 2007) and thorax (pectus carinatum, pectus excavatum or mixed) (Tocchioni et al. 2012).

In the preclinical and clinical stages of JH, hypermobile joints may be predisposed to an excess of macrotraumas and microtraumas. Macrotrauma includes luxations, subluxations, and injuries to soft tissues (muscles, ligaments, tendons, synovial membrane, and cartilage). Isolated or recurrent trauma due to excessive movement of the joints along non-physiological axes and aggravated by joint instability, can lead to acute pain and loss of function (Ericson and Wolman 2017; Nourissat et al. 2018). Microtrauma is a subtle, silent injury, typically unperceived by the individual, which may predispose to recurrent or persistent pain. This process can potentially lead to premature joint degeneration (also termed early osteoarthritis), which is the main cause of pain and disability in adults (Jasiewicz et al. 2010; Nourissat et al. 2018; Tibbo et al. 2019). Many of these manifestations are due to the fact that the diagnosis of JH in adults occurs without its recognition as an obvious generalized abnormality of the connective tissue and the cause of orthopaedic and rheumatological symptoms (Beighton et al. 2012).

The prevalence of JH is 2–57% in different populations (Remvig et al. 2007). It is common in childhood (Forléo et al. 1993; Lamari et al. 2005; León Ojeda and Castillo 2014; Lamari and Lamari 2016) and is found in 8–39% of schoolchildren (Rikken-Bultman et al. 1997). Nevertheless, the condition is underdiagnosed (Grahame 2013) and considered harmless by most healthcare providers (Hakim and Grahame 2003; Castori and Colombi 2015).

Consequences of Inadequate Postural Habits

As inadequate postural habits are repeated (Nowotny-Czupryna et al. 2013; O'Sullivan et al. 2017) and associated to the natural growth and maturation process of tissues (Matsudo et al. 1997; Ewertowska et al. 2020) such habits lead to structural manifestations by the end of the adolescent growth spurt (Sanders et al. 2017) predominantly due to changes in joint structure (Decker 2017; Chijimatsu and Saito 2019). These changes may include scoliosis and/or kyphoscoliosis (McMaster and Singh 1999; Newton et al. 2018) in the cervical (Munhoz et al. 2004; Priscila Weber et al. 2012; Kennedy et al. 2016) dorsal and lumbar (Richaud et al. 1990; Graup et al. 2010; Oliveira Pezzan et al. 2011; Jentzsch et al. 2017) regions. Potential physical abnormalities include pectus excavatum (Abid et al. 2017) pectus carinatum (Emil 2018) flat feet/valgus feet (Evans and Rome 2011; Cowie et al. 2012) valgus hallux (Mansur and Souza Nery 2020) genu recurvatum (Owens 2018; Dean et al. 2020) and temporomandibular disorders (Pasinato et al. 2011; Chang et al. 2018).

The gait may be affected, with internal rotation of the lower limbs in the majority of children with JH (Fig. 9.3) (Czamara et al. 2015). In a minority, the rotation of lower limbs is external, often with unilateral predominance. It is possible that postural habits are the cause of the unilateral predominance, with the weight load bearing on the medial aspect of the foot, which collapses, resulting in the straightening of the plantar arch. This process results in asymmetrical flat feet and places an excessive load on the hallux. The gait is abnormal and dysfunctional, in

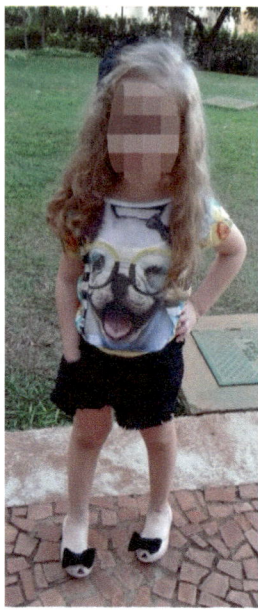

Fig. 9.3 Gait with internal rotation of the lower limbs

these circumstances, damage can occur to the knees, hips, and spine (Russek et al. 2019). These problems could be avoided by physiotherapeutic care in childhood (Lamari et al. 2022).

Children usually begin walking at an average age of 12 months (Chagas et al. 2020). However, the study conducted by Lamari et al. (2022) involving 482 individuals with JH in different age groups, showed a tendency toward delayed walking in those who did not crawl.

Hypermobility characteristics are perceptible in childhood by periodic evaluation of signs and symptoms which can be identified in the spine, limbs, and facial profile. The general lack of knowledge concerning JH can have a negative impact on these children, who miss the opportunity for early intervention. This situation explains why many adults with JH have physical disabilities stemming from a lack of timely interventions in childhood and/or adolescence. In turn, it changes the course of life of these individuals, with negative implications for social, recreational, sport, and occupational activities, as well as an impact on public funds (Lamari et al. 2022).

In 2005, Lamari et al. (2005) identified the need to adjust the Beighton scores (Beighton et al. 1973) for children due to the highly significant prevalence of scores ≥ 4 (64.6% of the 1120 children analysed). The authors pointed out the need for an adjustment of these scores, recognising the inconsistency between age groups. It is difficult to compare the results of studies that involved different age groups in the same sample with these same score parameters. Such conditions may often only be recognised when an affected individual is older and receives a secondary diagnosis.

References

Abid I, Ewais MM, Marranca J, Jaroszewski DE. Pectus excavatum: a review of diagnosis and current treatment options. J Am Osteopath Assoc. 2017;117:106–13.

Baeza-Velasco C, Sinibaldi L, Castori M. Attention-deficit/hyperactivity disorder, joint hypermobility-related disorders and pain: expanding body-mind connections to the developmental age. Atten Defic Hyperact Disord. 2018;10:163–75.

Bálint GP, Korda J, Hangody L, Bálint PV. Regional musculoskeletal conditions: foot and ankle disorders. Best Pract Res Clin Rheumatol. 2003;17:87–111.

Beighton P, Solomon I, Soskolne L. Articular mobility in an African population. Ann Rheum Dis. 1973;32:413–8.

Beighton P, Grahame R, Bird HA. Hypermobility of joints. 4th ed. London, UK: Springer; 2012.

Bravo JF. Síndrome de Ehlers-Danlos con especial énfasis en el síndrome de hiperlaxitud articular. Rev Med Chil. 2009;137:1488–97.

Castori M, Colombi M. Generalized joint hypermobility, JHsyndrome and Ehlers-Danlos syndrome, hypermobility type. Am J Med Genet C Semin Med Genet. 2015;169C:1–5.

Castori M, Hakim A. Contemporary approach to JHand related disorders. Curr Opin Pediatr. 2017;29:640–9.

Castori M, Morlino S, Pascolini G, Blundo C, Grammatico P. Gastrointestinal and nutritional issues in JHsyndrome/Ehlers-Danlos syndrome, hypermobility type. Am J Med Genet C Semin Med Genet. 2015;169C:54–75.

Chagas PSC, Fonseca ST, Santos TRT, Souza TR, Megale L, Silva PL, et al. Effects of baby walker use on the development of gait by typically developing toddlers. Gait Posture. 2020;76:231–7.

Chang CL, Wang DH, Yang MC, Hsu WE, Hsu ML. Functional disorders of the temporomandibular joints: Internal derangement of the temporomandibular joint. Kaohsiung J Med Sci. 2018;34:223–30.

Chijimatsu R, Saito T. Mechanisms of synovial joint and articular cartilage development. Cell Mol Life Sci. 2019;76:3939–52.

Chopra P, Tinkle B, Hamonet C, Brock I, Gompel A, Bulbena A, et al. Pain management in the Ehlers-Danlos syndromes. Am J Med Genet C Semin Med Genet. 2017;175:212–9.

Clavert P. Glenoid labrum pathology. Orthop Traumatol Surg Res. 2015;101(1 Suppl):S19–24.

Cowie S, Parsons S, Scammell B, McKenzie J. Hypermobility of the first ray in patients with planovalgus feet and tarsometatarsal osteoarthritis. Foot Ankle Surg. 2012;18:237–40.

Czamara A, Markowska I, Królikowska A, Szopa A, Domagalska SM. Kinematics of rotation in joints of the lower limbs and pelvis during gait: early results-SB ACLR approach versus DB ACLR approach. Biomed Res Int. 2015;2015:707168.

De León Ojeda NE, Castillo GD. Transtornos hereditários de la fibra colágena. Rev Cuba Hematol Inmunol Hemoter. 2014;30:405–7.

De Wandele I, Rombaut L, De Backer T, Peersman W, Da Silva H, De Mits S, et al. Orthostatic intolerance and fatigue in the hypermobility type of Ehlers-Danlos syndrome. Rheumatology (oxford). 2016;55:1412–20.

Dean RS, Graden NR, Kahat DH, DePhillipo NN, LaPrade RF. Treatment for symptomatic genu recurvatum: a systematic review. Orthop J Sports Med. 2020;8:2325967120944113.

Decker RS. Articular cartilage and joint development from embryogenesis to adulthood. Semin Cell Dev Biol. 2017;62:50–6.

El-Metwally A, Salminen JJ, Auvinen A, Macfarlane G, Mikkelsson M. Risk factors for development of non-specific musculoskeletal pain in preteens and early adolescents: a prospective 1-year follow-up study. BMC Musculoskelet Disord. 2007;8:46.

Emil S. Current options for the treatment of pectus Carinatum: when to brace and when to operate? Eur J Pediatr Surg. 2018;28:347–54.

Engelbert RH, Bank RA, Sakkers RJ, Helders PJ, Beemer FA, Uiterwaal CS. Pediatric generalized joint hypermobility with and without musculoskeletal complaints: a localized or systemic disorder? Pediatrics. 2003;111:e248–54.

Ericson WB Jr, Wolman R. Orthopaedic management of the Ehlers-Danlos syndromes. Am J Med Genet C Semin Med Genet. 2017;175:188–94.

Evans AM, Rome K. A Cochrane review of the evidence for non-surgical interventions for flexible pediatric flat feet. Eur J Phys Rehabil Med. 2011;47:69–89.

Ewertowska P, Trzaskoma Z, Sitarski D, Gromuł B, Haponiuk I, Czaprowski D. Muscle strength, muscle power and body composition in college-aged young women and men with Generalized Joint Hypermobility. PLoS ONE. 2020;15: e0236266.

Fatoye FO, Mosaku SK, Komolafe MA, Eegunranti BA, Adebayo RA, Komolafe EO, et al. Depressive symptoms and associated factors following cerebrovascular accident among Nigerians. JMH. 2009;18:224–32.

Forléo LH, Hilário MO, Peixoto AL, Naspitz C, Goldenberg J. Articular hypermobility in school children in Sao Paulo. Brazil J Rheumatol. 1993;20:916–7.

Gal-Nadasan N, Gal-Nadasan EG, Stoicu-Tivadar V, Poenaru DV, Popa-Andrei D. Measuring the negative impact of long sitting hours at high school students using the microsoft kinect. Stud Health Technol Inform. 2017;236:383–8.

Glans M, Bejerot S, Humble MB. Generalised JHand neurode-velopmental traits in a non-clinical adult population. B J Psych Open. 2017;3:236–42.

Godwin Y, Ter Horst B, Scerri G. Isolated Dorsoradial capsular tear of the thumb metacarpophalangeal joint: missed diagno-sis and the management of delayed presentation. Ann Plast Surg. 2018;80:121–4.

Goode AP, Cleveland RJ, Schwartz TA, Nelson AE, Kraus VB, Hillstrom HJ, et al. Relationship of JHwith low Back pain and lumbar spine osteoarthritis. BMC Musculoskelet Disord. 2019;20:158.

Grahame R. Joint hypermobility: emerging disease or illness behaviour? Clin Med (lond). 2013;13(Suppl 6):s50–2.

Grahame R, Hakim AJ. Hypermobility. Curr Opin Rheumatol. 2008;20:106–10.

Graup S, Santos SG, Moro ARP. Estudo descritivo de alter-ações posturais sagitais da coluna lombar em escolares da rede federal de ensino de Florianópolis. Rev Bras Ortop. 2010;45(5):453–9.

Gullo TR, Golightly YM, Flowers P, Jordan JM, Renner JB, Schwartz TA, et al. JHis not positively associated with prev-alent multiple joint osteoarthritis: a cross-sectional study of older adults. BMC Musculoskelet Disord. 2019;20:165.

Hakim AJ, Grahame R. A simple questionnaire to detect hyper-mobility: an adjunct to the assessment of patients with dif-fuse musculoskeletal pain. Int J Clin Pract. 2003;57:163–6.

Jasiewicz B, Potaczek T, Tesiorowski M, Lokas K. Spine deform-ities in patients with Ehlers-Danlos syndrome, type IV - late results of surgical treatment. Scoliosis. 2010;5:26.

Jentzsch T, Geiger J, König MA, Werner CM. Hyperlordosis is associated with facet joint pathology at the lower lumbar spine. Clin Spine Surg. 2017;30:129–35.

Junge T, Larsen LR, Juul-Kristensen B, Wedderkopp N. The extent and risk of knee injuries in children aged 9–14 with Generalised JHand knee JH- the CHAMPS-study Denmark. BMC Musculoskelet Disord. 2015;16:143.

Juul-Kristensen B, Johansen K, Hendriksen P, Melcher P, Sandfeld J, Jensen BR. Girls with generalized JHdisplay changed muscle activity and postural sway during static balance tasks. Scand J Rheumatol. 2016;45:57–65.

Kennedy BC, D'Amico RS, Youngerman BE, McDowell MM, Hooten KG, Couture D, et al. Long-term growth and alignment after occipitocervical and atlantoaxial fusion with rigid internal fixation in young children. J Neurosurg Pediatr. 2016;17:94–102.

Lamari NM, Lamari MM. Characterization of brazilian children with joint hypermobility. Int J Physiatry. 2016;2:011.

Lamari NM, Chueire AG, Cordeiro JA. Analysis of joint mobility patterns among preschool children. São Paulo Med J. 2005;123:119–23.

Lamari MM, Lamari NM, Medeiros MP, Pavarino EC. Signos y Síntomas en niños y adolescentes con Hipermovilidad Articular: Un estudio transversal cuantitativo observacional. Rev Chil Reumatol. 2020;36:42–53.

Lamari MM, Lamari NM, Araujo-Filho GM, Medeiros MP, Marques VRP, Pavarino EC. Psychosocial and motor characteristics of patients with hypermobility. Frontiers in Psychiatry. 2022. Frontiers in Psychiatry. https://doi.org/10.3389/fpsyt.2021.787822. 2022 Mar;12:787822.

Lui TH. Arthroscopy and endoscopy of the foot and ankle: indications for new techniques. Arthroscopy. 2007;23:889–902.

Mallorquí-Bagué N, Garfinkel SN, Engels M, Eccles JA, Pailhez G, Bulbena A, et al. Neuroimaging and psychophysiological investigation of the link between anxiety, enhanced affective reactivity and interoception in people with joint hypermobility. Front Psychol. 2014;5:1162.

Mansur NSB, Souza Nery CA. Hypermobility in hallux valgus. Foot Ankle Clin. 2020;25:1–17.

Marino LHC, Lamari N, Marino NW Jr. Hipermobilidade articular nos joelhos da criança. Arq Ciênc Saúde. 2004;11:124–7.

Matsudo SM, Paschoal VCP, Amancio OMS. Atividade Física e sua relação com o crescimento e a maturação biológica de crianças. Cad Nutr Soc Bras Aliment Nutr. 1997;14:1–12.

McMaster MJ, Singh H. Natural history of congenital kyphosis and kyphoscoliosis. A study of one hundred and twelve patients. J Bone Joint Surg Am. 1999;81:1367–83.

Mintz-Itkin R, Lerman-Sagie T, Zuk L, Itkin-Webman T, Davidovitch M. Does physical therapy improve outcome in infants with JHand benign hypotonia? J Child Neurol. 2009;24:714–9.

Mitakides J, Tinkle BT. Oral and mandibular manifestations in the Ehlers-Danlos syndromes. Am J Med Genet C Semin Med Genet. 2017;175:220–5.

Morris SL, O'Sullivan PB, Murray KJ, Bear N, Hands B, Smith AJ. Hypermobility and musculoskeletal pain in adolescents. J Pediatr. 2017;181:213-21.e1.

Munhoz WC, Marques AP, Siqueira JT. Radiographic evaluation of cervical spine of subjects with temporomandibular joint internal disorder. Braz Oral Res. 2004;18:283–9.

Newton PO, Kluck DG, Saito W, Yaszay B, Bartley CE, Bastrom TP. Anterior spinal growth tethering for skeletally immature patients with scoliosis: a retrospective look two to four years postoperatively. J Bone Joint Surg Am. 2018;100:1691–7.

Nourissat G, Vigan M, Hamonet C, Doursounian L, Deranlot J. Diagnosis of Ehlers-Danlos syndrome after a first shoulder dislocation. J Shoulder Elbow Surg. 2018;27:65–9.

Nowotny-Czupryna O, Czupryna K, Bąk K, Wróblewska E, Rottermund J. Postural habits of young adults and possibilities of modification. Ortop Traumatol Rehabil. 2013;15:9–21.

Oliveira Pezzan PA, João SM, Ribeiro AP, Manfio EF. Postural assessment of lumbar lordosis and pelvic alignment angles in adolescent users and nonusers of high-heeled shoes. J Manipulative Physiol Ther. 2011;34:614–21.

O'Sullivan P, Smith A, Beales D, Straker L. Understanding adolescent low back pain from a multidimensional perspective: implications for management. J Orthop Sports Phys Ther. 2017;47(10):741–51.

Owens BD. Recurvatum. Am J Sports Med. 2018;46:2833–5.

Palmer S, Bailey S, Barker L, Barney L, Elliott A. The effectiveness of therapeutic exercise for JHsyndrome: a systematic review. Physiotherapy. 2014;100:220–7.

Pasinato F, Souza JA, Corrêa EC, Silva AM. Temporomandibular disorder and generalized joint hypermobility: application of diagnostic criteria. Braz J Otorhinolaryngol. 2011;77:418–25.

Peterson B, Coda A, Pacey V, Hawke F. Physical and mechanical therapies for lower limb symptoms in children with hypermobility spectrum disorder and hypermobile Ehlers-danlos syndrome: a systematic review. J Foot Ankle Res. 2018;11:59.

Priscila Weber P, Corrêa ECR, Ferreira FS, Soares JC, Bolzan GP, Silva AMT. Cervical spine dysfunction signs and symptoms in individuals with temporomandibular disorder Frequência de sinais e sintomas de disfunção cervical em indivíduos com disfunção temporomandibular. J Soc Bras Fonoaudiol. 2012;24(2):134–9.

Remvig L, Jensen DV, Ward RC. Are diagnostic criteria for general JHand benign JHsyndrome based on reproducible and valid tests? A review of the literature. J Rheumatol. 2007;34:798–803.

Richaud J, Bousquet P, Ealet G, Clamens J, Beltchika K, Lazorthes Y. Recalibrage par voie postéro-latérale des sténoses traumatiques récentes du rachis dorsal et lombaire. Modalités et résultats à propos de 31 observations. Neurochirurgie 1990;36:27–38.

Rietveld AB. Dancers' and musicians' injuries. Clin Rheumatol. 2013;32:425–34.

Rikken-Bultman DG, Wellink L, van Dongen PW. Hypermobility in two Dutch school populations. Eur J Obstet Gynecol Reprod Biol. 1997;73:189–92.

Rombaut L, Malfait F, De Wandele I, Thijs Y, Palmans T, De Paepe A, et al. Balance, gait, falls, and fear of falling in women with the hypermobility type of Ehlers-Danlos syndrome. Arthritis Care Res (hoboken). 2011;63:1432–9.

Russek LN, Stott P, Simmonds J. Recognizing and effectively managing hypermobility-related conditions. Phys Ther. 2019;99:1189–200.

Sanders JO, Qiu X, Lu X, Duren DL, Liu RW, Dang D, et al. The uniform pattern of growth and skeletal maturation during the human adolescent growth spurt. Sci Rep. 2017;7:16705.

Scheper MC, Engelbert RH, Rameckers EA, Verbunt J, Remvig L, Juul-Kristensen B. Children with generalised JHand musculoskeletal complaints: state of the art on diagnostics, clinical characteristics, and treatment. Biomed Res Int. 2013;2013: 121054.

Scheper MC, Juul-Kristensen B, Rombaut L, Rameckers EA, Verbunt J, Engelbert RH. Disability adolescents and adults diagnosed with hypermobility-related disorders: a meta-analysis. Arch Phys Med Rehabil. 2016;97:2174–87.

Seçkin U, Tur BS, Yilmaz O, Yağci I, Bodur H, Arasil T. The prevalence of JHamong high school students. Rheumatol Int. 2005;25:260–3.

Simmonds JV, Keer RJ. Hypermobility and the hypermobility syndrome. Man Ther. 2007;12:298–309.

Sperotto F, Balzarin M, Parolin M, Monteforte N, Vittadello F, Zulian F. Joint hypermobility, growing pain and obesity are mutually exclusive as causes of musculoskeletal pain in schoolchildren. Clin Exp Rheumatol. 2014;32:131–6.

Tibbo ME, Wyles CC, Houdek MT, Wilke BK. Outcomes of primary total knee arthroplasty in patients with Ehlers-Danlos syndromes. J Arthroplasty. 2019;34:315–8.

Tocchioni F, Ghionzoli M, Pepe G, Messineo A. Pectus excavatum and MASS phenotype: an unknown association. J Laparoendosc Adv Surg Tech A. 2012;22:508–13.

Vařeková R, Vařeka I, Janura M, Svoboda Z, Elfmark M. Evaluation of postural asymmetry and gross joint mobility in elite female volleyball athletes. J Hum Kinet. 2011;29:5–13.

Wolf JM, Cameron KL, Owens BD. Impact of joint laxity and hypermobility on the musculoskeletal system. J Am Acad Orthop Surg. 2011;19:463–71.

Wong E, Altaf F, Oh LJ, Gray RJ. Adult degenerative lumbar scoliosis. Orthopedics. 2017;40:e930–9.

Yao Q, Wang S, Shin JH, Li G, Wood K. Motion characteristics of the lumbar spinous processes with degenerative disc disease and degenerative spondylolisthesis. Eur Spine J. 2013;22:2702–9.

10

Joint Hypermobility in Newborns and Children

Preclinical Stages of Joint Hypermobility in Newborns and Children

Throughout early childhood, up to 6 years of age, children can manifest musculoskeletal characteristics resulting from JH (Fig. 10.1). These features are insidious and become increasingly evident with the growth and maturation of tissues (Lamari et al. 2005, 2020; Stern et al. 2017; Lamari 2021).

These initial manifestations may or may not emerge, depending on the conditions that characterize each phase; not every individual with JH exhibits problems beginning in infancy. Determinants include gene penetrance and expression, which may differ between and even within families (Malfait et al. 2006; Morlino et al. 2017) as well as the infant's postural habits while sleeping and resting.

© The Author(s), under exclusive license to Springer Nature
Switzerland AG 2023
N. Lamari and P. Beighton, *Hypermobility in Medical Practice*,
In Clinical Practice, https://doi.org/10.1007/978-3-031-34914-0_10

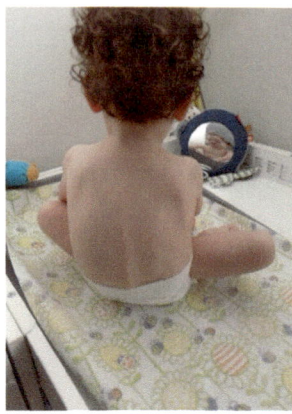

Fig. 10.1 The atypical positioning of the seated hypermobile child

Routine clinical practice shows that features related to JH are perceptible in most children. When manifested, impairments generally become greater throughout the different periods of life. Nevertheless, the majority are avoidable if identified early and the patient is referred for multidisciplinary care. It is important that emphasis is placed on physical therapy, as physical problems predominate (Terry et al. 2015; Engelbert et al. 2017; Lamari 2021).

Characteristics of Joint Hypermobility in Newborns

One of the first differences in newborns with JH characteristics is in the skin, which is unusually soft and silky. The sleep position may also differ from that of other neonates. Some infants may also exhibit mild to moderate hyper extensibility of the skin, which may be observed during a physical examination involving palpation (Engelbert et al. 2003; Malfait et al. 2020).

Newborns with JH may have inefficient sucking and frequent choking (Chatzoudis et al. 2015) with locomotor disorders, including difficulty holding their head a normal position, and inability to support the trunk adequately (Colloca and Polkinghorn 2003; Greenwood et al. 2011) due to weakness in the abdominal and paravertebral muscles (Fig. 10.2). Upper limb involvement follows and may be in the form of a weak grip, insufficient strength to sustain the body in the "cat" position. Subluxations and/or luxations in the upper limbs, especially the shoulders may occur (Sosnoff et al. 2007; Kaya et al. 2015). For these reasons, affected children either do not crawl or crawl in an unusual way (Lamari et al. 2021).

Joint instability in the ankles and toes (Latey et al. 2017; Whelan et al. 2019) is a visible characteristic that also differentiates these children from other newborns. Some have unstable knees, with possible episodes of subluxation/luxation of the patella (Beighton et al. 2012; Hasler and Studer 2017; Jaquith and Parikh 2017; Lamari et al. 2020).

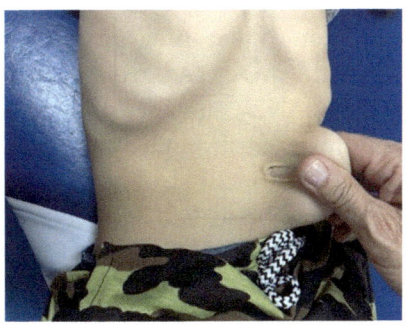

Fig. 10.2 Increased skin elasticity in child

Delays in neuropsychomotor development stages are evident in early childhood due to ankle instability, flat feet, clumsiness and coordination disorders (Hasler and Studer 2017). Walking may be either early or delayed, depending on the extent of JH in the upper and/or lower limbs. These children may have difficulty in supporting their head, arms, trunk, and legs, with delayed, absent, or altered crawling partially due to weakness in the arms (Caram et al. 2006; Piedimonte et al. 2018).

This weakness may hinder the crawling phase or enable only atypical crawling, such as dragging the gluteus muscles with assistance of the legs. Moreover, weakness in the legs leads to delayed walking due to instability in the hips, knees and/or ankles, especially if their hand grip is too weak to assist in standing (Lamari 2021).

Atypical postures are evident when holding an affected newborn. When the condition predominates in the upper limbs, there is a tendency to maintain the arms loose ("tired shoulders") due to difficulty in supporting the upper limbs. In such instances, there is a risk of shoulder and elbow luxation. In the sitting up phase or when held in the lap, these children may have difficulty maintaining the trunk erect, as hypermobility is present in the trunk, with consequent insufficiency of the soft tissues of the back and abdominal region.

In this condition, there is a predominance of the forward lean of the head and trunk; sitting with the vertebral axis in concavity, shoulder protrusion, and atypical abdominal protrusion (rounded sitting) in contrast to other newborns (Lamari 2021). A tendency to maintain this posture into adulthood leads to the development of deformities in the thorax and vertebral axis (Milhorat et al. 2007).

Other variable characteristics in affected neonates include chest deformity (Kurkov et al. 2018) protruding ears (Bravo 2009) deformity in one or more fingers and/ or toes (Olshan et al. 2003; Ejjiyar and Ettalbi 2018) club-foot (Olshan et al. 2003; Beck et al. 2010) and/or muscular torticollis (Kuo et al. 2014). The skin of the feet may show premature aging or broad and/or widely spaced and/or asymmetrical and/or large or small toes. The ears may be protruded, normal or small in size, with very small asymmetrical lobes (Stembridge et al. 2015; Martiniuk et al. 2017). There may be abdominal hernias (Kelly and Ponsky 2013; Cevik et al. 2014) with a greater frequency of abdominal diastasis (Oetgen et al. 2017; Vilanova-Sánchez et al. 2017) and umbilical hernia (Fig. 10.3) (McNair et al. 2006; Burcharth et al. 2015; Conner et al. 2018). It is possible that some of these abnormalities result

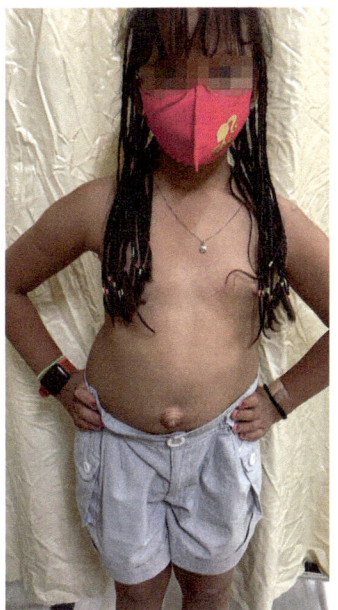

Fig. 10.3 Umbilical hernia in the child with JH

from impaired neurological factors occurring while the fetus is in the uterus.

Newborns with JH may have congenital abnormalities in the head shape (Tollefson 2016) or asymmetry of the face (Karacan et al. 2019; Launonen et al. 2019) which are suggestive of repetitive head postures in intrauterine life (Beuriat et al. 2019). An abnormal head shape and facial asymmetry after childbirth is suggestive of a repetitive head posture in lateral or dorsal decubitus while lying in bed, with the maintenance of improper head postures due to the impaired neuromuscular impulses. These children are often regarded by their parents as a "quiet baby".

In clinical practice, many of the affected children are considered as having neurological sequelae, while the real problem may be a benign motor dysfunction of a musculoskeletal origin due to JH. A small proportion of these children have temporary or permanent motor and cognitive sequelae. This situation may lead to secondary diagnoses that have consequences for the patient and family throughout the different periods of life.

References

Beck JJ, Nazif MA, Sangiorgio SN, Semel JI, Ebramzadeh E, Zionts LE. Does generalized joint hypermobility influence the Ponseti treatment of clubfoot patients? J Pediatr Orthop B. 2010;30:66–70.

Beighton P, Grahame R, Bird HA. Hypermobility of joints, 4th ed. London, UK: Springer, 2012;5:65–94.

Beuriat PA, Szathmari A, Di Rocco F, Mottolese C. Deformational plagiocephaly: State of the art and review of the literature. Neurochirurgie. 2019;65:322–9.

Bravo JF. Síndrome de Ehlers-Danlos con especial énfasis en el síndrome de hiperlaxitud articular. Rev Med Chil. 2009;137:1488–97.

Burcharth J, Pedersen MS, Pommergaard HC, Bisgaard T, Pedersen CB, Rosenberg J. The prevalence of umbilical and epigastric hernia repair: a nationwide epidemiologic study. Hernia. 2015;19:815–9.

Caram LH, Funayama CA, Spina CI, Giuliani LR, Pina Neto JM. Investigação das causas de atraso no neurodesenvolvimento: recursos e desafios. Arq Neuropsiquiatr. 2006;64:466–72.

Cevik M, Yazgan P, Aksoy N. Evaluation of antioxidative/oxidative status and prolidase parameters in cases of inguinal hernia with joint hypermobility syndrome. Hernia. 2014;18:849–53.

Chatzoudis D, Kelly TJ, Lancaster J, Jones TM. Upper airway obstruction in a patient with Ehlers-Danlos syndrome. Ann R Coll Surg Engl. 2015;97:e50–1.

Colloca CJ, Polkinghorn BS. Chiropractic management of Ehlers-Danlos syndrome: a report of two cases. J Manipulative Physiol Ther. 2003;26:448–59.

Conner P, Vejde JH, Burgos CM. Accuracy and impact of prenatal diagnosis in infants with omphalocele. Pediatr Surg Int. 2018;34:629–33.

Ejjiyar M, Ettalbi S. Complex management of macrodactylia of the hand: between aesthetic and functional prejudice. Pan Afr Med J. 2018;30:45.

Engelbert RH, Bank RA, Sakkers RJ, Helders PJ, Becmer FA, Uiterwaal CS. Pediatric generalized joint hypermobility with and without musculoskeletal complaints: a localized or systemic disorder? Pediatrics. 2003;111:e248–54.

Engelbert RH, Juul-Kristensen B, Pacey V, de Wandele I, Smeenk S, Woinarosky N, et al. The evidence-based rationale for physical therapy treatment of children, adolescents, and adults diagnosed with joint hypermobility syndrome/hypermobile Ehlers Danlos syndrome. Am J Med Genet C Semin Med Genet. 2017;175:158–67.

Greenwood NL, Duffell LD, Alexander CM, McGregor AH. Electromyographic activity of pelvic and lower limb muscles during postural tasks in people with benign joint hypermobility syndrome and non hypermobile people. A Pilot Study Man Ther. 2011;16:623–8.

Hasler CC, Studer D. Patella instability in children and adolescents. EFORT Open Rev. 2017;1:160–6.

Jaquith BP, Parikh SN. Predictors of Recurrent Patellar Instability in Children and Adolescents After First-time Dislocation. J Pediatr Orthop. 2017;37:484–90.

Karacan K, Sabancıoğulları V, Koşar MI, Karacan A. The effect of the functional asymmetry of the brain on face morphometry in the university students of mathematics and painting department. Folia Morphol (warsz). 2019;78:508–16.

Kaya P, Alemdaroğlu İ, Yılmaz Ö, Karaduman A, Topaloğlu H. Effect of muscle weakness distribution on balance in neuromuscular disease. Pediatr Int. 2015;57:92–7.

Kelly KB, Ponsky TA. Pediatric abdominal wall defects. Surg Clin North Am. 2013;93:1255–67.

Kuo AA, Tritasavit S, Graham JM Jr. Congenital muscular torticollis and positional plagiocephaly. Pediatr Rev. 2014;35:79–87.

Kurkov AV, Paukov VS, Fayzullin AL, Shekhter AB. Costal cartilage changes in children with pectus excavatum and pectus carinatum. Arkh Patol. 2018;80:8–15.

Lamari NM, Chueire AG, Cordeiro JA. Analysis of joint mobility patterns among preschool children. São Paulo Med J. 2005;123:119–23.

Lamari MM, Lamari NM, Medeiros MP, Pavarino EC. Signos y Síntomas en niños y adolescentes con Hipermovilidad Articular: Un estudio transversal cuantitativo observacional. Rev Chil Reumatol. 2020;36:42–53.

Lamari NM, Baeza-Velasco C, Araújo Filho GM, Lamari MM, Medeiros MP. Transtorno do espectro do autismo e síndrome de Ehlers-Danlos - tipo hipermobilidade: um relato de caso. Arch Health Sci. 2021;28(1):46–8.

Lamari MM. Apresentação fenotípica das condições relacionadas aos transtornos de hipermobilidade em diferentes fases da vida [tese]. São José do Rio Preto: Faculdade de Medicina de São José do Rio Preto; 2021.

Latey PJ, Burns J, Hiller CE, Nightingale EJ. Relationship between foot pain, muscle strength and size: a systematic review. Physiotherapy. 2017;103:13–20.

Launonen AM, Vuollo V, Aarnivala H, Heikkinen T, Pirttiniemi P, Valkama AM, et al. Craniofacial Asymmetry from One to Three Years of Age: A Prospective Cohort Study with 3D Imaging. J Clin Med 2019;9(1):70.

Malfait F, Hakim AJ, De Paepe A, Grahame R. The genetic basis of the joint hypermobility syndromes. Rheumatology (oxford). 2006;45:502–7.

Malfait F, Castori M, Francomano CA, Giunta C, Kosho T, Byers PH. The Ehlers-Danlos syndromes. Nat Rev Dis Primers. 2020;6:64.

Martiniuk AL, Vujovich-Dunn C, Park M, Yu W, Lucas BR. Plagiocephaly and Developmental Delay: A Systematic Review. J Dev Behav Pediatr. 2017;38:67–78.

McNair C, Hawes J, Urquhart H. Caring for the newborn with an omphalocele. Neonatal Netw. 2006;25:319–27.

Milhorat TH, Bolognese PA, Nishikawa M, McDonnell NB, Francomano CA. Syndrome of occipitoatlantoaxial hypermobility, cranial settling, and chiari malformation type I in patients with hereditary disorders of connective tissue. J Neurosurg Spine. 2007;7:601–9.

Morlino S, Dordoni C, Sperduti I, Venturini M, Celletti C, Camerota F, et al. Refining patterns of joint hypermobility, habitus, and orthopedic traits in joint hypermobility syndrome and Ehlers-Danlos syndrome, hypermobility type. Am J Med Genet A. 2017;173:914–29.

Oetgen ME, Andelman S, Martin BD. Age-Based Normative Measurements of the Pediatric Pelvis. J Orthop Trauma. 2017;31:e205–9.

Olshan AF, Schroeder JC, Alderman BW, Mosca VS. Joint laxity and the risk of clubfoot. Birth Defects Res A Clin Mol Teratol. 2003;67:585–90.

Piedimonte C, Penge R, Morlino S, Sperduti I, Terzani A, Giannini MT, et al. Exploring relationships between joint hypermobility and neurodevelopment in children (4–13 years) with hereditary connective tissue disorders and developmental coordination disorder. Am J Med Genet B Neuropsychiatr Genet. 2018;177:546–56.

Sosnoff JJ, Deutsch KM, Newell KM. Does muscular weakness account for younger children's enhanced force variability? Dev Psychobiol. 2007;49:399–405.

Stembridge NS, Vandersteen AM, Ghali N, Sawle P, Nesbitt M, Pollitt RC, et al. Clinical, structural, biochemical and X-ray crystallographic correlates of pathogenicity for variants in the C-propeptide region of the COL3A1 gene. Am J Med Genet A. 2015;167A:1763–72.

Stern CM, Pepin MJ, Stoler JM, Kramer DE, Spencer SA, Stein CJ. Musculoskeletal Conditions in a Pediatric Population with Ehlers-Danlos Syndrome. J Pediatr. 2017;181:261–6.

Terry RH, Palmer ST, Rimes KA, Clark CJ, Simmonds JV, Horwood JP. Living with joint hypermobility syndrome: patient experiences of diagnosis, referral and self-care. Fam Pract. 2015;32:354–8.

Tollefson TT. Congenital Deformities of the Face, Head, and Neck. Facial Plast Surg. 2016;32:121–2.

Vilanova-Sánchez A, Ching CB, Gasior AC, Diefenbach K, Wood RJ, Levitt M. Image of the Month: Clinical Features in a Newborn with Covered Cloacal Exstrophy. European J Pediatr Surg Rep. 2017;5(1):e57–9.

Whelan AJ, Tolaymat A, Rainey SC. Bumbling, Stumbling, Fumbling: Weakness, Steppage Gait, and Facial Droop in a 3-Year-Old Male. Glob Pediatr Health 2019;6:2333794X19865858.

11

Joint Hypermobility in Children, Preadolescents and Adolescents

Preclinical and Clinical Manifestations of Joint Hypermobility in Children, Preadolescents and Adolescents

The period of preadolescence (10–14 years of age) is the most important phase for the definitive development of the structures and functioning of the locomotor apparatus (Inocencio Arocena et al. 2004; Schmidt et al. 2017) facial profile, and oral health (Fig. 11.1) (Coster et al. 2005; Jensen and Storhaug 2012; Mitakides and e Tinkle 2017; Lamari et al. 2020). Thus, this period has implications for most adults with joint hypermobility (JH) sequelae because their tissues are less robust.

These individuals are sometimes guided in preadolescence by healthcare providers who might be unaware or only marginally familiar with the manifestations of JH. For this reason, the opportunity for timely preventive and

© The Author(s), under exclusive license to Springer Nature Switzerland AG 2023
N. Lamari and P. Beighton, *Hypermobility in Medical Practice*,
In Clinical Practice, https://doi.org/10.1007/978-3-031-34914-0_11

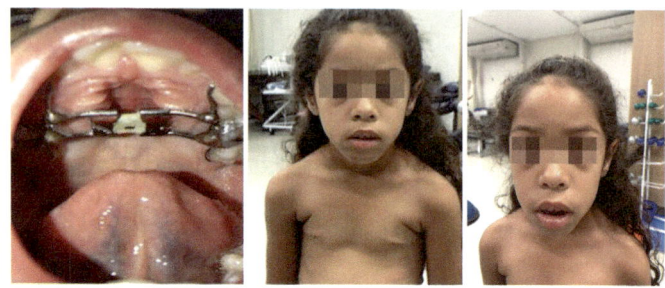

Fig. 11.1 Aesthetic and functional impairment of oral health and facial profile

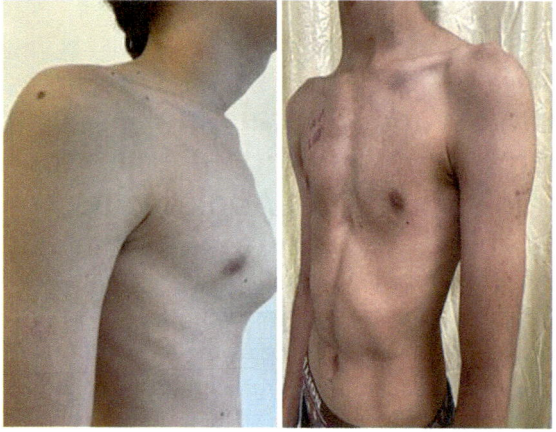

Fig. 11.2 Thoracic deformity in two hypermobile adolescents boys

corrective interventions could be lost. Indeed, this period passes very quickly. Actions demand knowledge regarding the body patterns of this population in each stage of life for the identification of preclinical manifestations, such as signs and symptoms in the spine, chest, limbsand facial profile (Fig. 11.2).

In adolescence, which ranges from 15 to 19 years of age, most individuals have already gone through the growth spurt (Sheehy et al. 2000; Soliman et al. 2014). Most adolescents with hypermobile joints have physical sequelae due to the lack of an early detection of the underlying structural characteristics (Schmidt et al. 2017; Bukva et al. 2019; Lamari et al. 2020). In this period, clinical manifestations may emerge, including orthopedic problems involving the spine (Fig. 11.3) (Czaprowski 2014; Stern et al. 2016; Ericson and Wolman 2017) and lower limbs (Berglund et al. 2005; Evans and Rome 2011; Ross et al. 2011) arthralgia (Jacome 1999; Kerr et al. 2000; Castori et al. 2015; Ericson and Wolman 2017) neuralgia (Hamonet 2013; Daniels et al. 2016; Ericson and Wolman 2017) fatigue (Murray et al. 2013; Hakim et al. 2017a) and difficulty in sleeping (Hakim et al. 2017a).

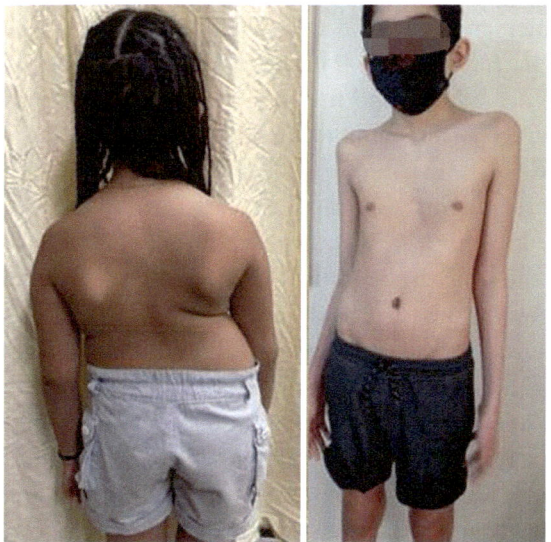

Fig. 11.3 Scoliosis in the children with JH

Preclinical and Clinical Characteristics in Preadolescents with Joint Hypermobility

There is importance in observation of static and dynamic physical postures and poor postural habits (Booshanam et al. 2011; Lisi et al. 2020) during activities of daily living. Instrumental, recreational, and sport activities throughout this period are also important, especially between 10 and 14 years of age. This phase includes the growth spurt, which occurs in a five-year period in both sexes (eight to 13 years of age for girls and 10–15 years of age for boys) (Morlino et al. 2017; Carrascosa et al. 2018) In this period, the structures of the locomotor apparatus are defined and preclinical signs of structural deformities may be observed. The outcome of treatment is influenced by the period of evolution, severity, and timing of the interventions (Wolf et al. 2011; Schmidt et al. 2017). The characteristics of JH have often been noticed by parents since infancy and may not be valued by pediatricians. However, it is possible to identify preclinical signs in this period.

Most patients seek physiotherapy due to issues related to the locomotor apparatus (back, limbs and facial profile) after the growth spurt. In this period structural changes and deformities are already defined for adulthood, altering the course of the individual's physical health (Danielsson and Hallerman 2015; Negrini et al. 2015).

A recent study of hypermobile children in South America confirmed that musculoskeletal and extraskeletal (systemic) manifestations were frequent in children and preadolescents with JH. Most had psychosocial concerns, joint pain, and other manifestations affecting the skin, feet, and face. Approximately half of affected individuals had joint pain, especially in the lower limbs, and a history of "growing pains", such as stomach pain, gastrointestinal and neurological disorders, delayed acquisition of gait, sleep disorders, and fatigue (Lamari et al. 2020). In view of this wide range of abnormalities it is important to recognise JH. Population-based studies are needed to correlate these manifestations in children and adolescents with JH based on the new criteria for HSDs and hEDS (Lamari et al. 2020).

Preclinical and Clinical Characteristics in Adolescents with Joint Hypermobility

Most adolescents with JH, when seeking assistance, have already gone through the growth spurt period (Sheehy et al. 2000; Soliman et al. 2014) with rare exceptions (Gasser et al. 2001; Carrascos et al. 2018). In this period, clinical manifestations emerge with structural deformities of the locomotor apparatus. Many individuals with JH are believed to have functional and/or structural impairments, as it is unlikely that they have been submitted to specific interventions (Lamari et al. 2020). Sequelae can be identified in these adolescents (Schmidt et al. 2017; Bukva et al. 2019). In contrast, those submitted to programs for the prevention of structural changes are less likely to have problems stemming from the poor use of body mechanics.

Adolescence is a phase of important physical and physiological changes that are manifested in a more intense manner (Machado et al. 2009). The identification of JH features in children underscores the need for studies involving adolescents. This is a period in which the definitive body posture of the adult is established and with it

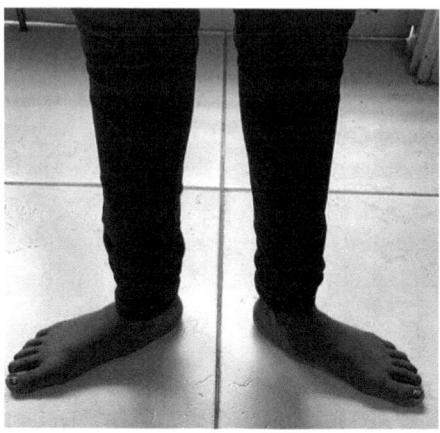

Fig. 11.4 Flat feet in an adolescent with JH

come the several problems that imply limitations and back pain, which affect approximately 80% of the population at some point in life (Andersson 2003; Ehrlich 2003; Kääriä et al. 2005). The knees are involved in most affected individuals due to hyperextension (Myer et al. 2008) and the consequent degenerative processes in this joint (Simpson 2006).

Orthopedic manifestations commonly found in individuals with JH, include kyphosis (Ericson and Wolman 2017) scoliosis (Stanitski et al. 2000; Adib et al. 2005; Czaprowski 2014; Stern et al. 2016) flat feet (Fig. 11.4) (Berglund et al. 2005; Evans and Rome 2011; Ross et al. 2011) and genu recurvatum (Marino et al. 2004). Oral and mandibular structural changes are also found in the soft tissues of the mouth and dentition, along with facial pain, headache, and altered functioning of the temporomandibular joints (Mitakides and e Tinkle 2017). Arthralgias (Kerr et al. 2000; Ericson and Wolman 2017) and neuralgias (Daniels et al. 2016; Ericson and Wolman 2017) may also occur. In this context of unawareness of the implications for the locomotor apparatus, adolescents with JH often suffer frequent, successive injuries that can exert an impact in adulthood, leading to a reduction in quality of life (Mu et al. 2019).

Joint laxity can cause harm to health (Grahame 2016; Ericson and Wolman 2017) and is followed by degenerative processes (Ericson and Wolman 2017) and reductions in muscle strength and endurance, exerting a negative impact on quality of life (Landry et al. 2015). Affected people often have pain (Maeland et al. 2011; Murray et al. 2013; Hamonet et al. 2015; Chopra et al. 2017) such as chronic headaches, which are frequent and vary in type and severity (Jacome 1999; Castori et al. 2015) contributing to the disability (Rombaut et al. 2010, 2012). The entire body has been described as painful since early childhood (Hamonet 2013). Moreover, fibromyalgia is a common concomitant condition (Ting et al. 2012) and is strongly associated with sleep disorders, including abnormal sleep architecture (Hakim et al. 2017b).

Fatigue has a multifactorial etiology and occurs in most adolescents with JH. This condition emerges as a persistent sensation of weariness, a lack of energy and exhaustion, which has a negative impact on concentration. Contributing factors are pain, sleep disorders, dysautonomia, allergies, and/or medications (Hakim et al. 2017a). These patients report trouble with sleeping, including insomnia and non-restorative sleep. Several other factors can also affect sleep, such as pain, dysautonomia, poor sleep hygiene, and medications (Murray et al. 2013; Hakim et al. 2017a).

Although some individuals with JH may reach adolescence without any structural deformities, they are still exposed due to their frail, hypermobile joints, especially during sport and recreational activities due to an unawareness of their problem and the inherent risks (Sanches et al. 2015). The "Parkour" sport is an example of a radical sport modality that requires body skills that few possess (Nicholson et al. 2017; Wright et al. 2020) and practitioners of this sport are exposed to accidents (Schwarz et al. 1993; Rombaut et al. 2011) It has been suggested that adolescents who practice Parkour may have hypermobile joints and are unaware of their condition. They are at risk of suffering injuries due to their frailer tissues and joint disability (Junge et al. 2015; Schmidt et al. 2017; Bukva et al. 2019).

Beginning with the growth spurt period, negative impacts can be experienced in scholastic, recreational, sport, and professional activities, with the "exception" of some who benefit from hypermobility, such as contortionists, dancers, athletes, pianists and violinists (Duren et al. 2013; Malina et al. 2013; Soliman et al. 2014) Nevertheless, these individuals are also negatively affected due to the inadequate repetitive forces exerted on their frail tissues.

A large number of studies have been undertaken on JH. However, there is a need for more in-depth research, as the differentiation between hypermobile and non-hypermobile individuals is not yet well defined. Equally, there is no consensus on the optimum degree of mobility for the promotion of physical health. In Brazil, investigations of the peculiarities of this condition are needed given the country's geographic size, its different climates, distinct sociocultural attributes, and diversified colonization (Lamari et al. 2020).

References

Adib N, Davies K, Grahame R, Woo P, Murray KJ. Joint hypermobility syndrome in childhood. A not so benign multisystem disorder? Rheumatology (Oxford) 2005;44:744–50.

Andersson GBJ. Epidemiological features of chronic low-back pain. Lancet 1999;354:581–5.

Berglund B, Nordström G, Hagberg C, Mattiasson AC. Foot pain and disability in individuals with Ehlers-Danlos syndrome (EDS): impact on daily life activities. Disabil Rehabil. 2005;27:164–9.

Booshanam DS, Cherian B, Joseph CP, Mathew J, Thomas R. Evaluation of posture and pain in persons with benign joint hypermobility syndrome. Rheumatol Int. 2011;31:1561–5.

Bukva B, Vrgoč G, Madić DM, Sporiš G, Trajković N. Correlation between hypermobility score and injury rate in artistic gymnastics. J Sports Med Phys Fitness. 2019;59:330–4.

Carrascosa A, Yeste D, Moreno-Galdó A, Gussinyé M, Ferrández Á, Clemente M, et al. Crecimiento puberal de 1.453 niños sanos según la edad de inicio de la pubertad. Estudio longitudinal de Barcelona. An Pediatr (Barc) 2018;89:144–52.

Castori M, Morlino S, Ghibellini G, Celletti C, Camerota F, Grammatico P. Connective tissue, Ehlers-Danlos syndrome(s), and head and cervical pain. Am J Med Genet C Semin Med Genet. 2015;169C:84–96.

Chopra P, Tinkle B, Hamonet C, Brock I, Gompel A, Bulbena A, et al. Pain management in the Ehlers-Danlos syndromes. Am J Med Genet C Semin Med Genet. 2017;175:212–9.

Czaprowski D. Generalised joint hypermobility in caucasian girls with idiopathic scoliosis: relation with age, curve size, and curve pattern. Scientific World J. 2014;2014:1–6.

Daniels AH, DePasse JM, Kamal RN. Orthopaedic surgeon burnout: diagnosis, treatment, and prevention. J Am Acad Orthop Surg. 2016;24:213–9.

Danielsson AJ, Hallerman KL. Quality of life in middle-aged patients with idiopathic scoliosis with onset before the age of 10 years. Spine Deform. 2015;3:440–50.

De Coster PJ, Martens LC, De Paepe A. Oral health in prevalent types of Ehlers-Danlos syndromes. J Oral Pathol Med. 2005;34:298–307.

Duren DL, Seselj M, Froehle AW, Nahhas RW, Sherwood RJ. Skeletal growth and the changing genetic landscape during childhood and adulthood. Am J Phys Anthropol. 2013;150:48–57.

Ericson WB Jr, Wolman R. Orthopaedic management of the Ehlers-Danlos syndromes. Am J Med Genet C Semin Med Genet. 2017;175:188–94.

Evans AM, Rome K. A Cochrane review of the evidence for non-surgical interventions for flexible pediatric flat feet. Eur J Phys Rehabil Med. 2011;47:69–89.

Ehrlich GE. Low back pain. Bull World Health Organ. 2003;81:671–6.

Gasser T, Sheehy A, Molinari L, Largo RH. Growth of early and late matures. Ann Hum Biol. 2001;28:328–36.

Grahame R. Ehlers-Danlos syndrome. S Afr Med J. 2016;106(6 Suppl 1):S45–6.

Hakim A, Wandele I, O'callaghan C, Pocinki A, Rowe P. Chronic fatigue in Ehlers-Danlos syndrome-hypermobile type. Am J Med Genet C Semin Med Genet. 2017a;175:175–80.

Hakim A, O'Callaghan C, De Wandele I, Stiles L, Pocinki A, Rowe P. Cardiovascular autonomic dysfunction in Ehlers-Danlos syndrome-Hypermobile type. Am J Med Genet C Semin Med Genet. 2017b;175:168–74.

Hamonet C. Les douleurs dans le syndrome d'Ehlers-Danlos (à propos de 644 cas avec un test de Beighton égal ou supérieur à 4/9). J Réadaptation Médicale. 2013;33:51–3.

Hamonet C, Gompel A, Mazaltarine G, Brock I, Baeza-Velasco C, Zeitoun JD, et al. Ehlers-Danlos syndrome or disease? J Syndromes. 2015;2:5.

Inocencio Arocena J, Ocaña Casas I, Benito OL. Laxitud articular: prevalencia y relación con dolor musculosquelético. An Pediatr (barc). 2004;61:162–6.

Jacome DE. Headache in Ehlers-Danlos syndrome. Cephalalgia. 1999;19:791–6.

Jensen JL, Storhaug K. Dental implants in patients with Ehlers-Danlos syndrome: a case series study. Int J Prosthodont. 2012;25:60–2.

Junge T, Larsen LR, Juul-Kristensen B, Wedderkopp N. The extent and risk of knee injuries in children aged 9–14 with Generalised Joint Hypermobility and knee joint hypermobility - the CHAMPS-study Denmark. BMC Musculoskelet Disord. 2015;16:143.

Kääriä S, Kaila-Kangas L, Kirjonen J, Riihimäki H, Luukonen R, Leino-Arjas P. Low back pain, work absenteeism, chronic back disorders, and clinical findings in the low back as predictors of hospitalization due to low back disorders: a 28-year follow-up of industrial employees. Spine. 2005;30:1211–8.

Kerr A, Macmillan CE, Uttley WS, Luqmani RA. Physiotherapy for children with hypermobility syndrome. Physiotherapy. 2000;86:313–7.

Lamari MM, Lamari NM, Medeiros MP Pavarino EC. Signos y Síntomas en niños y adolescentes con Hipermovilidad Articular: Un estudio transversal cuantitativo observacional. Rev Chil Reumatol. 2020;36:42–53.

Landry BW, Fischer PR, Driscoll SW, Koch KM, Harbeck-Weber C, Mack KJ, et al. Managing chronic pain in children and adolescents: a clinical review. PM R. 2015;7(Suppl 11):S295-315.

Lisi C, Monteleone S, Tinelli C, Rinaldi B, Di Natali G, Savasta S. Postural analysis in a pediatric cohort of patients with Ehlers-Danlos Syndrome: a pilot study. Minerva Pediatr. 2020;72:73–8.

Machado DRL, Bonfim MR, Costa LT. Pico de velocidade de crescimento como alternativa para classificação aturacional associada ao desempenho motor. Rev Bras Cineantropom Desemp Hum. 2009;11(1):14–21.

Maeland S, Assmus J, Berglund B. Subjective health complaints in individuals with Ehlers Danlos syndrome: a questionnaire study. Int J Nurs Stud. 2011;48:720–4.

Malina RM, Baxter-Jones AD, Armstrong N, Beunen GP, Caine D, Daly RM, et al. Role of intensive training in the growth and maturation of artistic gymnasts. Sports Med. 2013;43:783–802.

Marino LHC, Lamari N, Marino NW Jr. Hipermobilidade articular nos joelhos da criança. Arq Ciênc Saúde. 2004;11:124–7.

Mitakides J e Tinkle BT. Oral and mandibular manifestations in the ehlers–danlos syndromes. Am J Med Genet C Semin Med Genet. 2017;175:220–225.

Morlino S, Dordoni C, Sperduti I, Venturini M, Celletti C, Camerota F, et al. Refining patterns of joint hypermobility, habitus, and orthopedic traits in joint hypermobility syndrome and Ehlers-Danlos syndrome, hypermobility type. Am J Med Genet A. 2017;173:914–29.

Mu W, Muriello M, Clemens JL, Wang Y, Smith CH, Tran PT, et al. Factors affecting quality of life in children and adolescents with hypermobile Ehlers-Danlos syndrome/hypermobility spectrum disorders. Am J Med Genet A. 2019;179:561–9.

Murray B, Yashar BM, Uhlmann WR, Clauw DJ, Petty EM. Ehlers-Danlos syndrome, hypermobility type: a characterization of the patients' lived experience. Am J Med Genet A. 2013;161A:2981–8.

Myer GD, Ford KR, Paterno MV, Nick TG, Hewett TE. The effects of generalized joint laxity on risk of anterior cruciate ligament injury in young female athletes. Am J Sports Med. 2008;36:1073–80.

Negrini S, Minozzi S, Bettany-Saltikov J, Chockalingam N, Grivas TB, Kotwicki T, et al. Braces for idiopathic scoliosis in adolescents. Cochrane Database Syst Rev. 2015;(6):CD006850.

Nicholson LL, Adams RD, Tofts L, Pacey V. Physical and psychosocial characteristics of current child dancers and non-dancers with systemic joint hypermobility: a descriptive analysis. J Orthop Sports Phys Ther. 2017;47:782–91.

Rombaut L, Malfait F, Cools A, De Paepe A, Calders P. Musculoskeletal complaints, physical activity and health related quality of life among patients with the Ehlers-Danlos syndrome hypermobility type. Disabil Rehabil. 2010;32:1339–45.

Rombaut L, Malfait F, De Paepe A, Rimbaut S, Verbruggen G, De Wandele I, et al. Impairment and impact of pain in female patients with Ehlers-Danlos syndrome: a comparative study with fibromyalgia and rheumatoid arthritis. Arthritis Rheum. 2011;63:1979–87.

Rombaut L, Malfait F, De Wandele I, Mahieu N, Thijs Y, Segers P, et al. Muscle-tendon tissue properties in the hypermobility type of Ehlers-Danlos syndrome. Arthritis Care Res (hoboken). 2012;64:766–72.

Ross A, Hauser MD, Phillips HJ. Treatment of joint hypermobility syndrome, including Ehlers-Danlos syndrome, with Hackett-Hemwall Prolotherapy. J Prolotherapy. 2011;3:612–29.

Sanches SB, Oliveira GM, Osório FL, Crippa JA, Martín-Santos R. Hypermobility and joint hypermobility syndrome in Brazilian students and teachers of ballet dance. Rheumatol Int. 2015;35:741–7.

Schmidt H, Pedersen TL, Junge T, Engelbert R, Juul-Kristensen B. Hypermobility in adolescent athletes: pain, functional ability, quality of life, and musculoskeletal injuries. J Orthop Sports Phys Ther. 2017;47:792–800.

Schwarz N, Ohner T, Schwarz AF, Gerschpacher M, Meznik A. Injuries of the cervical spine in children and adolescents. Unfallchirurg. 1993;96(5):235–41.

Sheehy A, Gasser T, Molinari L, Largo RH. Contribution of growth phases to adult size. Ann Hum Biol. 2000;27:281–98.

Simpson MR. Benign joint hypermobility syndrome: evaluation, diagnosis, and management. J Am Osteopath Assoc. 2006;106:531–6.

Soliman A, De Sanctis V, Elalaily R, Bedair S. Advances in pubertal growth and factors influencing it: can we increase pubertal growth? Indian J Endocrinol Metab. 2014;18(Suppl 1):S53–62.

Stanitski DF, Nadjarian R, Stanitski CL, Bawle E, Tsipouras P. Orthopaedic manifestations of Ehlers-Danlos syndrome. Clin Orthop. 2000;376:213–21.

Stern CM, Pepin MJ, Stoler JM, Kramer DE, Spencer SA, Stein CJ. Musculoskeletal conditions in a pediatric population with Ehlers-Danlos syndrome. J Pediatr. 2016;181:261–6.

Ting TV, Hashkes PJ, Schikler K, Desai AM, Spalding S, Kashikar-Zuck S. The role of benign joint hypermobility in the pain experience in juvenile fibromyalgia: an observational study. Pediatr Rheumatol Online J. 2012;10:16.

Wolf JM, Cameron KL, Owens BD. Impact of joint laxity and hypermobility on the musculoskeletal system. J Am Acad Orthop Surg. 2011;19:463–71.

Wright KE, Furzer BJ, Licari MK, Dimmock JA, Jackson B, Thornton AL. Exploring associations between neuromuscular performance, hypermobility, and children's motor competence. J Sci Med Sport. 2020;23:1080–5.

12

Joint Hypermobility in Adults

Clinical Manifestations, Habits and Posture in Adults with Joint Hypermobility

Young adults with a history of joint hypermobility (JH) may have outcomes resulting from initial signs and symptoms that probably emerged in childhood and/or adolescence. In adulthood, these individuals may seek a diagnosis and treatment for the various manifestations that have resulted in functional disabilities and/or physical disabilities. Most of these problems arose in the growth spurt period, in association with poor postural habits during static and dynamic activities, these include placement of the body in the sitting, lying, or standing position, or during movement. These problems stem from less robust tissues that are insufficient to support the diversity of body positions and are greater and more apparent in adulthood.

© The Author(s), under exclusive license to Springer Nature Switzerland AG 2023
N. Lamari and P. Beighton, *Hypermobility in Medical Practice*, In Clinical Practice, https://doi.org/10.1007/978-3-031-34914-0_12

In elderly people with hypermobility, structural changes may occur in the locomotor apparatus, facial profile, and oral health. Other problems include subluxations, with physical disability and chronic pain, are mainly due to progressive, anti-functional osteoarticular deformities. These complications may also occur due to the maturation of tissues with changes in the composition and conformation of joint extremities.

Early identification of each musculoskeletal signs and symptoms in childhood and/or adolescence could significantly contribute to changing the course of the health-disease process in this JH population.

Habits and Postural Attitudes in Clinical Stages of Current or Past Joint Hypermobility in Young Adults

Young adults with JH may have had progressive musculoskeletal deformities and extra-skeletal manifestations since childhood. Lack of early care can lead to adults with both structural and functional physical sequelae (Fig. 12.1).

Esthetic and functional changes may be found in the facial profile, oral health, spine, and limbs. The facial profile may have features such as a triangular face, thin nose, deviated septum, protruding ears, myopia, blue sclera and astigmatism. There may be dental crowding, protrusion of the dental arch (Mitakides and Tinkle 2017; Lamari et al. 2020) and mouth breathing (Jensen and Storhaug 2012; Lamari et al. 2020). There may be scoliosis, genu recurvatum, fallen arches, valgus hallux, and edema in the extremities. The upper limbs may be "soft" and the hands may have the "flying bird" sign (Simsek et al. 2019; Tinkle and Levy 2019; Lamari et al. 2020). These manifestations

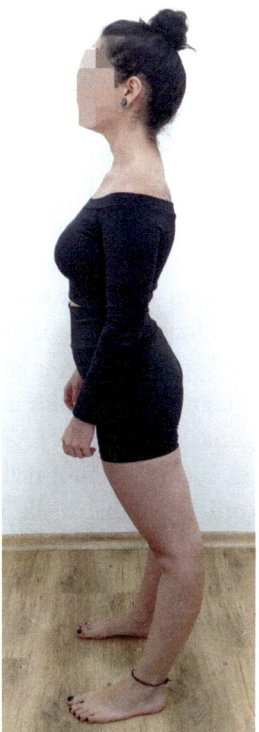

Fig. 12.1 Postural pattern of adults with JH

are always dependent on the penetrance and expression of the determinant gene (Castori and Colombi 2015).

The upper and lower limbs may show muscle weakness and joint luxations or subluxations, with greater frequency in the shoulders and/or knees (Tobias et al. 2013). Specific characteristics may occur, such as hyperextension of the elbows and/or knees, hyperflexion and/or hyperextension of the wrists and/or ankles. Inadequate, involuntary postural features of the fingers and/or toes and scapulae may determine joint deformities in these regions, with negative effects on the esthetics of static and dynamic posture (King and Toolan 2004; Celletti et al. 2012).

Cumulative injuries involving inflammatory processes as a response to trauma, including osteoarthritis and tendinitis, with the wear of per-articular and intra-articular structures (Flowers et al. 2018; Goode et al. 2019; Tinkle 2020). These may have a negative impact on occupations, sports, and daily activities and they can be accompanied by psychological and/or psychiatric problems (Baeza-Velasco et al. 2011; Bulbena et al. 2017).

In routine clinical practice, young adults may seek diagnosis and treatment of articular and extra articular manifestations (Ilgunas et al. 2020). The most frequent secondary diagnoses include, fibromyalgia, osteoarthritis, herniated cervical and/or lumbar disk, flat feet, tendinitis, and emotional disorders (Sendur et al. 2007).

A firm diagnosis provides a sense of well-being and better understanding on the part of families and healthcare providers, as well as a better understanding in school, recreational, sports, and work settings. Many seek medical assistance due to musculoskeletal pain (Lamari et al. 2020) such as chondromalacia, herniated disk and osteoarthritis. Those for whom no abnormalities are found on imaging often receive a diagnosis of fibromyalgia or diagnoses related to psychological or psychiatric aspects of their condition (Gedalia et al. 1993; Goldman 2001; Sendur et al. 2007; Baeza-Velasco et al. 2011; Bulbena et al. 2017).

There is difficulty occurs in recognizing JH in undiagnosed adults, as the process of aging modifies the configuration of joint extremities, as well as the peri- and intra-articular soft tissues (Dolan et al. 2003; Brown et al. 2011; Quarrier 2011). In turn, this further hinders the diagnosis of the primary disorder by functional physical examination. This situation places a burden on the healthcare system and exerts a negative impact on the quality of life of these individuals in all phases of life. There are also negative implications for their families. In this context it is relevant that the true prevalence of JH in the community is unknown (Beighton et al. 2012).

Orthopedic complications are common, with the frequent occurrence of luxations or pain in the shoulders and knees, together with problems with the heels and iliotibial band syndrome (Tobias et al. 2013). Kyphosis is a common finding in individuals with EDS and occurs due to the loose ligament structures, and poor postural habits (Ericson and Wolman 2017). Scoliosis is also common in the EDS (Mack 2010; Stern et al. 2016). Low muscle strength, poor endurance, impaired functional performance, an increase in fatigue, and diminished quality of life are frequent in affected persons (Landry et al. 2015). It would be appropriate for surgical interventions to be delayed until all non surgical options have been exhausted (Weinberg et al. 1999; Daniels et al. 2016).

Musculoskeletal conditions have been identified in 30% (Connelly et al. 2015) to 55% (Clark and Simmonds 2011) of adults with JH in outpatient care. These problems are often attributed to excessive movement and inadequate muscle control. In the feet, many of the differences in mechanics and control between normal feet and flat feet have not been quantified (Hunt and Smith 2004). Valgus foot in children can be classified as flexible or rigid (Cass and Camasta 2010; Pothrat et al. 2013). Hypermobility in the foot is a common finding, but difficult to quantify. Primary tarsometatarsal arthritis is less common and has an uncertain etiology, but there is a greater range of motion than that found in normal feet. Investigation into this association could lead to progress in both prevention and treatment (Cowie et al. 2012).

Flat feet can exert a significant negative impact on activities of daily living, such as less propulsion capacity and a less functional gait (Jankowicz-Szymanska et al. 2013; Galli et al. 2014). Individuals with EDS have mobility difficulties due to problems with the feet and consequent functional disability. It is therefore important to assess foot status and seek solutions for walking problems, which could have an impact on affected individual's quality of life (Berglund et al. 2005).

JH is not always painful. Nevertheless, pain can occur prior to the emergence of radiographic findings. Individuals with unidentified EDS can develop premature joint wear, which results in a higher failure rate of clinical and surgical treatment (Ericson and Wolman 2017).

Awareness of the association between hypermobility and musculoskeletal injuries is important in the avoidance of these problems. Long-term therapy and general conditioning may be needed, with an emphasis on improving strength and proprioception. Recognition of the implications of JH is crucial in the management and rehabilitation of musculoskeletal injuries and associated orthopedic conditions (Wolf et al. 2011).

Clinical Manifestations of Articular Hypermobility in Elderly Individuals

Common manifestations of JH in elderly affected individuals include deformities of the spine, shoulders, hands, knees, ankles, and feet. These include scoliosis, kyphoscoliosis, and osteoarthritis of the hips, knees, fingers, and toes (Fig. 12.2) (Jasiewicz et al. 2010; Nourissat et al. 2018; Tibbo et al. 2019). Many affected persons may have had hip replacement surgery (Naal et al. 2017; Uemura et al. 2017) and interventions targeting the knees (Wang

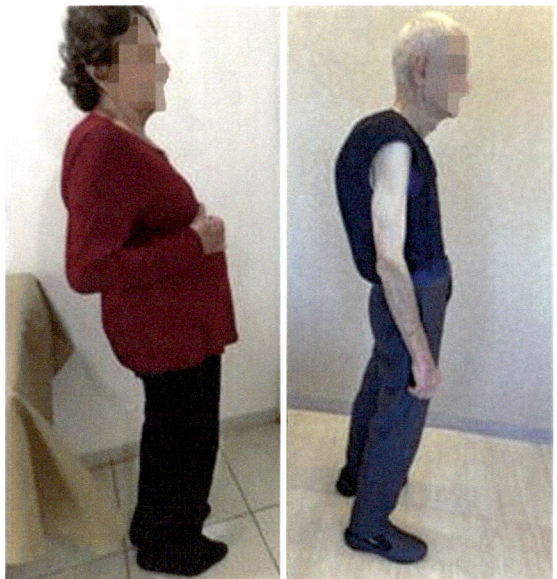

Fig. 12.2 Postural pattern of elderly people with JH

et al. 2018) and shoulders (Mangano et al. 2016; Fram et al. 2019) Others have had surgical intervention for the correction of flat feet, valgus foot, and valgus hallux (Fig. 12.3). It is possible to prevent or treat the manifestations of all these complications if they are detected early, preferably in childhood (Castori and Hakim 2017; O'Sullivan et al. 2017).

Chronic musculoskeletal symptoms in elderly adults may lead to the conclusion that they progressively lost their features of GJH due to the process of aging. This situation may also have a negative impact on joint range of motion in individuals with JH. For these reasons, a five-point questionnaire was created as a screening tool to investigate the history of JH in this age group (Hakim and Grahame 2003). This assessment tool has made a significant contribution to research and clinical practice.

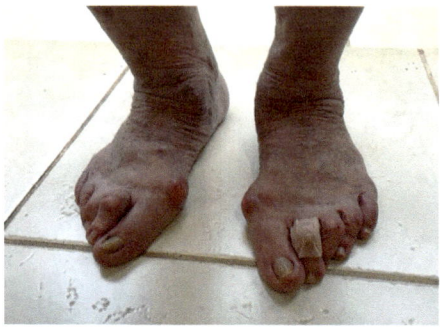

Fig. 12.3 Hallux valgus deformities in an elderly woman with JH

References

Baeza-Velasco C, Gély-Nargeot MC, Bulbena Vilarrasa A, Bravo JF. Joint hypermobility syndrome: problems that require psychological intervention. Rheumatol Int. 2011;31:1131–6.

Beighton P, Grahame R, Bird HA. Hypermobility of joints. 4th ed. London, UK: Springer, 2012;5:65–94.

Berglund B, Nordström G, Hagberg C, Mattiasson AC. Foot pain and disability in individuals with Ehlers-Danlos syndrome (EDS): impact on daily life activities. Disabil Rehabil. 2005;27:164–9.

Brown JC, Miller CJ, Schwellnus MP, Collins M. Range of motion measurements diverge with increasing age for COL5A1 genotypes. Scand J Med Sci Sports. 2011;21:e266–72.

Bulbena A, Baeza-Velasco C, Bulbena-Cabré A, Pailhez G, Critchley H, Chopra P, et al. Psychiatric and psychological aspects in the Ehlers-Danlos syndromes. Am J Med Genet C Semin Med Genet. 2017;175:237–45.

Cass AD, Camasta CA. A review of tarsal coalition and pes planovalgus: clinical examination, diagnostic imaging, and surgical planning. J Foot Ankle Surg. 2010;49:274–93.

Castori M, Hakim A. Contemporary approach to joint hypermobility and related disorders. Curr Opin Pediatr. 2017;29:640–9.

Castori M, Colombi M. Generalized joint hypermobility, joint hypermobility syndrome and Ehlers-Danlos syndrome, hypermobility type. Am J Med Genet C Semin Med Genet. 2015;169C:1–5.

Celletti C, Castori M, Grammatico P, Camerota F. Evaluation of lower limb disability in joint hypermobility syndrome. Rheumatol Int. 2012;32:2577–81.

Clark CJ, Simmonds JV. An exploration of the prevalence of hypermobility and joint hypermobility syndrome in Omani women attending a hospital physiotherapy service. Musculoskeletal Care. 2011;9:1–10.

Connelly E, Hakim A, Davenport HS, Simmonds JV. A Study exploring the prevalence of Hypermobility Syndrome in a musculoskeletal triage clinic. Physiother Res Pract. 2015;36:43–53.

Cowie S, Parsons S, Scammell B, McKenzie J. Hypermobility of the first ray in patients with planovalgus feet and tarsometatarsal osteoarthritis. Foot Ankle Surg. 2012;18:237–40.

Daniels AH, DePasse JM, Kamal RN. Orthopaedic surgeon burnout: diagnosis, treatment, and prevention. J Am Acad Orthop Surg. 2016;24:213–9.

Dolan AL, Hart DJ, Doyle DV, Grahame R, Spector TD. The relationship of joint hypermobility, bone mineral density, and osteoarthritis in the general population: the Chingford Study. J Rheumatol. 2003;30:799–803.

Ericson WB Jr, Wolman R. Orthopaedic management of the Ehlers-Danlos syndromes. Am J Med Genet C Semin Med Genet. 2017;175:188–94.

Flowers PPE, Cleveland RJ, Schwartz TA, Nelson AE, Kraus VB, Hillstrom HJ, et al. Association between general joint hypermobility and knee, hip, and lumbar spine osteoarthritis by race: a cross-sectional study. Arthritis Res Ther. 2018;20:76.

Fram B, Elder A, Namdari S. Periprosthetic humeral fractures in shoulder arthroplasty. JBJS Rev. 2019;7(11): e6.

Galli M, Cimolin V, Rigoldi C, Pau M, Costici P, Albertini G. The effects of low arched feet on foot rotation during gait in children with down syndrome. J Intellect Disabil Res. 2014;58:758–64.

Gedalia A, Press J, Klein M, Buskila D. Joint hypermobility and fibromyalgia in schoolchildren. Ann Rheum Dis. 1993;52:494–6.

Goldman JA. Fibromyalgia and hypermobility. J Rheumatol. 2001;28:920–1.

Goode AP, Cleveland RJ, Schwartz TA, Nelson AE, Kraus VB, Hillstrom HJ, et al. Relationship of joint hypermobility with low Back pain and lumbar spine osteoarthritis. BMC Musculoskelet Disord. 2019;20:158.

Hakim A, Grahame R. Joint hypermobility. Best Pract Res Clin Rheumatol. 2003;17:989–1004.

Hunt AE, Smith RM. Mechanics and control of the flat versus normal foot during the stance phase of walking. Clin Biomech (bristol, Avon). 2004;19:391–7.

Ilgunas A, Wänman A, Strömbäck M. "I was cracking more than everyone else": young adults' daily life experiences of hypermobility and jaw disorders. Eur J Oral Sci. 2020;128:74–80.

Jankowicz-Szymanska A, Mikolajczyk E, Wojtanowski W. The effect of the degree of disability on nutritional status and flat feet in adolescents with down syndrome. Res Dev Disabil. 2013;34:3686–90.

Jasiewicz B, Potaczek T, Tesiorowski M, Lokas K. Spine deformities in patients with Ehlers-Danlos syndrome, type IV - late results of surgical treatment. Scoliosis. 2010;5:26.

Jensen JL, Storhaug K. Dental implants in patients with Ehlers-Danlos syndrome: a case series study. Int J Prosthodont. 2012;25:60–2.

King DM, Toolan BC. Associated deformities and hypermobility in hallux valgus: an investigation with weightbearing radiographs. Foot Ankle Int. 2004;25:251–5.

Lamari MM, Lamari NM, Medeiros MP, Pavarino EC. Signos y Síntomas en niños y adolescentes con Hipermovilidad Articular: Un estudio transversal cuantitativo observacional. Rev Chil Reumatol. 2020;36:42–53.

Landry BW, Fischer PR, Driscoll SW, Koch KM, Harbeck-Weber C, Mack KJ, et al. Managing chronic pain in children and adolescents: A clinical review PM R 2015;7 Suppl 11:S295-315.

Mack KJ. Management of chronic daily headache in children. Expert Rev Neurother. 2010;10:1479–86.

Mangano T, Cerruti P, Repetto I, Felli L, Ivaldo N, Giovale M. Reverse shoulder arthroplasty in older patients: is it worth it? A subjective functional outcome and quality of life survey. Aging Clin Exp Res. 2016;28:925–33.

Mitakides J, Tinkle BT. Oral and mandibular manifestations in the Ehlers-Danlos syndromes. Am J Med Genet C Semin Med Genet. 2017;175:220–5.

Naal FD, Müller A, Varghese VD, Wellauer V, Impellizzeri FM, Leunig M. Outcome of Hip Impingement Surgery: does Generalized Joint Hypermobility Matter? Am J Sports Med. 2017;45:1309–14.

Nourissat G, Vigan M, Hamonet C, Doursounian L, Deranlot J. Diagnosis of Ehlers-Danlos syndrome after a first shoulder dislocation. J Shoulder Elbow Surg. 2018;27:65–9.

O'Sullivan P, Smith A, Beales D, Straker L. Understanding adolescent low back pain from a multidimensional perspective: implications for management. J Orthop Sports Phys Ther. 2017;47:741–51.

Pothrat C, Authier G, Viehweger E, Rao G. Multifactorial gait analysis of children with flat foot and hind foot valgus deformity. Comput Methods Biomech Biomed Engin. 2013;16(Suppl 1):80–1.

Quarrier NF. Is hypermobility syndrome (HMS) a contributing factor for chronic unspecific wrist pain in a musician? If so, how is it evaluated and managed? Work. 2011;40:325–33.

Sendur OF, Gurer G, Bozbas GT. The frequency of hypermobility and its relationship with clinical findings of fibromyalgia patients. Clin Rheumatol. 2007;26:485–7.

Simsek IE, Elvan A, Selmani M, Cakiroglu MA, Kirmizi M, Bayraktar BA, et al. Generalized hypermobility syndrome (GHS) alters dynamic plantar pressure characteristics. J Back Musculoskelet Rehabil. 2019;32:321–7.

Stern CM, Pepin MJ, Stoler JM, Kramer DE, Spencer SA, Stein CJ. Musculoskeletal conditions in a pediatric population with Ehlers-Danlos syndrome. J Pediatr. 2016;181:261–6.

Tibbo ME, Wyles CC, Houdek MT, Wilke BK. Outcomes of primary total knee arthroplasty in patients with Ehlers Danlos syndromes. J Arthroplasty. 2019;34:315–8.

Tinkle BT. Symptomatic joint hypermobility. Best Pract Res Clin Rheumatol. 2020;34: 101508.

Tinkle BT, Levy HP. Symptomatic joint hypermobility: the hypermobile type of Ehlers-Danlos syndrome and the hypermobility spectrum disorders. Med Clin North Am. 2019;103:1021–33.

Tobias JH, Deere K, Palmer S, Clark EM, Clinch J. Joint hypermobility is a risk factor for musculoskeletal pain during adolescence: findings of a prospective cohort study. Arthritis Rheum. 2013;65:1107–15.

Uemura K, Takao M, Otake Y, Koyama K, Yokota F, Hamada H, et al. Change in pelvic sagittal inclination from supine to standing position before hip arthroplasty. J Arthroplasty. 2017;32:2568–73.

Wang W, Yang K, Yang P, Song D, Wang C, Song J, et al. Primary total knee arthroplasty for complex supracondylar femoral fractures in patients with knee arthritis: a retrospective study of a patient cohort. Medicine (baltimore). 2018;97: e12700.

Weinberg J, Doeriing C, McFarland EG. Joint surgery in Ehlers-Danlos patients: results of a survey. Am J Orthop. 1999;28:406–9.

Wolf JM, Cameron KL, Owens BD. Impact of joint laxity and hypermobility on the musculoskeletal system. J Am Acad Orthop Surg. 2011;19:463–71.

13

Physiotherapy for Joint Hypermobility Disorders

Promotion, Prevention, and Rehabilitation of Joint Hypermobility-Related Conditions

Diagnostic support and treatments provided by different specialties that address hypermobile Ehlers-Danlos syndrome (hEDS), hypermobility spectrum disorders (HSD), and joint hypermobility syndrome (JHS) are important in the management of problems inherent in joint hypermobility (JH). It is relevant that persons with these conditions often seek treatment for several different problems at the same time. In addition, the early diagnosis of hEDS/HSD/JHS also enables the monitoring and management of possible comorbidities (Gensemer et al. 2021).

Physiotherapeutic care is essential for individuals with asymptomatic JH and/or JH disorders of the locomotor system, whether involving deformities, pain, trauma,

© The Author(s), under exclusive license to Springer Nature Switzerland AG 2023
N. Lamari and P. Beighton, *Hypermobility in Medical Practice*,
In Clinical Practice, https://doi.org/10.1007/978-3-031-34914-0_13

muscle dysfunction, inadequate postural habits, ergonomic inadequacies, preparation for daily physical activities, sports, and instrumental, recreational, or occupational activities. Physical therapy aims at health promotion, disability prevention and physical-functional rehabilitation. It is well recognised that less robust tissues, muscle weakness, biomechanical changes and joint subluxation/dislocation often manifest predominantly as joint and muscle pain (Fig. 13.1) (Grahame 2009; Beighton et al. 2012; Engelbert et al. 2017).

Children can experience multiple disabilities as a result of increased connective tissue laxity, with complications including pain (Ferrell et al. 2004; Adib et al. 2005; Kemp et al. 2010; Pacey et al. 2015; Scheper et al. 2016), joint instability (Shirley et al. 2012; Scheper et al. 2016), extra-articular factors (Kort et al. 2003; Adib et al. 2005; Kirby and Davies 2007; Pacey et al. 2015), and psychological symptoms (Fatoye et al. 2012; Mu et al. 2018; Baeza-Velasco et al. 2019). Impaired development of motor activity, gait pattern, physical fitness and (Adib et al. 2005; Kirby et al. 2005; Kirby and Davies 2007; Mintz-Itkin et al. 2009; Falkerslev et al. 2013) participation in recreation, sports and social activities (Jansson et al. 2004; Adib et al. 2005; Schubert-Hjalmarsson et al. 2012; Birt et al. 2014) are other relevant factors.

Pain relief is a clear objective for persons with hypermobility conditions and, although the use of chronic pain medication(s) has shown some success, most are not very effective (Younger et al. 2014). The use of medication(s) does not alter the cause of pain, which may be exacerbated due to the high incidence of gastroesophageal problems in these disorders (Castori et al. 2012). A thorough knowledge of gastrointestinal presentations and their management is therefore necessary for the avoidance of morbidity or even mortality (Solomon et al. 1996; Castori

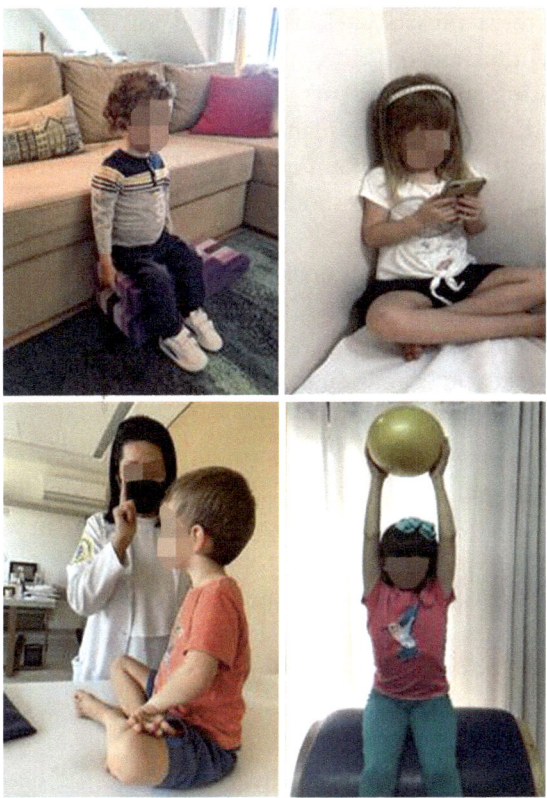

Fig. 13.1 Physiotherapeutic assistance in ergonomic adequacy and for trunk stabilization in children with JH

et al. 2015). It is important that on-surgical options for treating joint pain should be attempted before recommending surgery (Grahame 2009; Daniels et al. 2016).

Exercise is essential for pain relief (Engelbert et al. 2017). In physical therapy, daily exercises involving strength training and others that address proprioception, joint stability, and control of extreme ranges of motion are beneficial (Gensemer et al. 2021). Low-impact, isometric and eccentric strengthening exercises are effective for chronic musculoskeletal pain and for improving proprioception and posture, increasing muscle strength and stabilising specific joints such as the spine, shoulder and knee (Ericson and Wolman 2017). Nevertheless, physical exercises that expose joints to the risk of dislocations and manipulative therapies should be used carefully (Gensemer et al. 2021).

Orthoses are occasionally recommended for unstable joints, including those in the limbs and spine. Finger, wrist, knee and ankle stabilisers and cervical collars may also be useful (Simmonds and Keer 2008; Ericson and Wolman 2017; Hamonet 2018). The utility of protocols for the use of orthoses has been emphasised. Appropriate management can be extremely helpful in relieving pain by stabilising specific joints. Nevertheless, overuse can weaken muscles.

Children with stretched or lax ligaments may experience delayed motor development (Adib et al. 2005) with difficult postural control resulting from excessive joint movement (Fig. 13.2) (Galli et al. 2011). These children may require physical therapy to stimulate neuro-psycho-motor development, most often to support the head and trunk but also to roll, crawl, walk, run and jump. This motor impairment may manifest as difficulties in playing with other children, resulting in social exclusion. For this reason early physical therapy interventions are essential during the school-age period to improve school performance and mitigate socialisation losses. Both of these factors have implications for the quality of life of the child and family.

Proprioceptive acuity is necessary to maintain joint stability at all ages (Fig. 13.3); however, it is impaired in persons with hEDS/HSD/JHS. Knee joint stability may be impaired and it is frequently related to the development of osteoarthritis (Clayton et al. 2015). Further studies

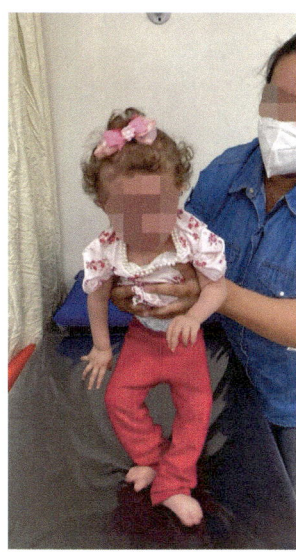

Fig. 13.2 Mother of child with motor delay being trained for activities at home

are necessary for the understanding of the relationship between the joint(s), proprioception, and osteoarthritis, and/or the extent to which these problems are acquired or inherited (Beighton et al. 2012). The implementation of a proprioceptive training programme should focus on the knee, including hyperextension, because it is less stable due to muscle weakness and proprioception disorders (Fatoye et al. 2011). Abnormal and non-physiological gait patterns are due to the biomechanical consequences of JH and may lead to an increased frequency of falls (Galli et al. 2011).

Decreased proprioception is usually present in symptomatic patients (Smith et al. 2013) who have muscle weakness (Rombaut et al. 2012; Scheper et al. 2016). Reduced proprioception and muscle strength significantly interact and can generate increasing limitations to the activities of

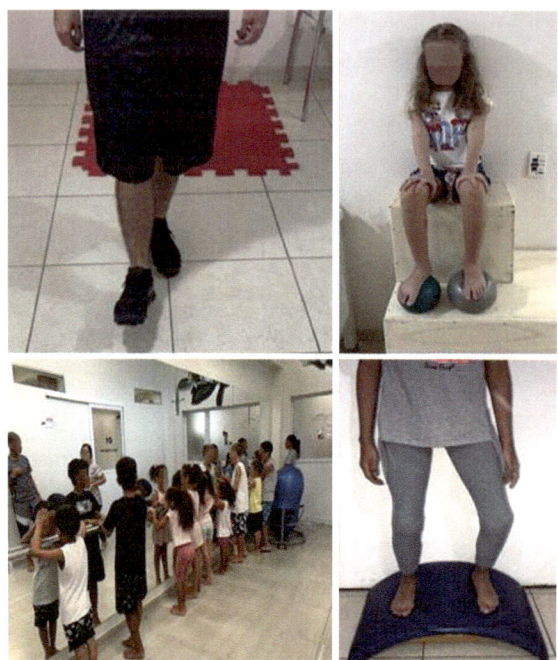

Fig. 13.3 Physical therapy assistance in proprioceptive training

daily living and negatively influence motor performance. There is suggestive evidence supporting a significant association between generalised JH and developmental coordination disorders (Ghibellini et al. 2015). The coexistence of these conditions warrants consideration in rehabilitation planning (Scheper et al. 2016).

Physical therapy approaches should prioritise training of the patient and informing the parents of the possible implications of a JH condition on locomotor system mechanics. Thus, it is important to understand the mechanisms used to stabilise the joints in a static and dynamic manner and in the standing, sitting, and lying (i.e., prone and supine) positions. This concept is applicable to different activities and age groups. Depending on the purpose of physical therapy, the regimen will be defined for a specified period. This period will include daily care or on specific days because there are differences in patient's activities, with specific clinical variations among different age groups.

Treatment requires multidisciplinary cooperation. Periodic consultations may be necessary for diagnostic support and treatment from cardiologists, orthopaedic surgeons, oral and maxillofacial surgeons, gastroenterologists, and ophthalmologists, among others (Gazit et al. 2016). Complex symptoms are often present and may pose a challenge to effective professional management.

Modification of the collagen extracellular matrix probably plays an important role in the impairment of the mechanical stability of affected tissues in patients with the EDS. These changes probably feedback into the cells, resulting in altered mechanical sensitisation and the cell phenotype. In this way, the propagation of mechanical, cellular, and physiological changes may result in chronic disease responses and lead to tissue damage and instability. Stabilisation of the modified extracellular matrix environment can establish positive mechanical signals that can reverse cellular and physiological phenotypes and yield long-term benefits. This fact highlights the need for careful physical therapy for connective tissues which are already compromised (Gensemer et al. 2021).

References

Adib N, Davies K, Grahame R, Woo P, Murray KJ. Joint hypermobility syndrome in childhood. A not so benign multisystem disorder? Rheumatology (Oxford) 2005;44(6):744–50.

Baeza-Velasco C, Bulbena A, Polanco-Carrasco R, Jaussaud R. Cognitive, emotional, and behavioral considerations for chronic pain management in the Ehlers-Danlos syndrome hypermobility-type: a narrative review. Disabil Rehabil. 2019;41(9):1110–8. https://doi.org/10.1080/09638288.201 7.1419294. Epub 2018 Jan 22.

Beighton P, Grahame R, Bird H. Hypermobility of joints. 4th ed. London: Springer; 2012.

Birt L, Pfeil M, MacGregor A, Armon K, Poland F. Adherence to home physiotherapy treatment in children and young people with joint hypermobility: a qualitative report of family perspectives on acceptability and efficacy. Musculoskeletal Care. 2014;12:56–61.

Castori M, Morlino S, Ghibellini G, Celletti C, Camerota F, Grammatico P. Connective tissue, Ehlers-Danlos syndrome(s), and head and cervical pain. Am J Med Genet C Semin Med Genet. 2015;169C:84–96.

Castori M, Morlino S, Celletti C, Celli M, Morrone A, Colombi M, et al. Management of pain and fatigue in the joint hypermobility syndrome (a.k.a. Ehlers-Danlos syndrome, hypermobility type): principles and proposal for a multidisciplinary approach. Am J Med Genet A 2012;158A:2055–70.

Clayton HA, Jones SAH, Henriques DYP. Proprioceptive precision is impaired in Ehlers-Danlos syndrome. Springerplus. 2015;4(1):1–8. https://doi.org/10.1186/s40064-015-1089-1.

Daniels AH, DePasse JM, Kamal RN. Orthopaedic surgeon burnout: diagnosis, treatment, and prevention. J Am Acad Orthop Surg. 2016;24:213–9.

De Kort LM, Verhulst JA, Engelbert RH, Uiterwaal CS, de Jong TP. Lower urinary tract dysfunction in children with generalized hypermobility of joints. J Urol. 2003;170:1971–4.

Engelbert RH, Juul-Kristensen B, Pacey V, de Wandele I, Smeenk S, Woinarosky N, et al. The evidence-based rationale for physical therapy treatment of children, adolescents, and adults diagnosed with joint hypermobility syndrome/

hypermobile Ehlers Danlos syndrome. Am J Med Genet C Semin Med Genet. 2017;175:158–67.

Ericson WB Jr, Wolman R. Orthopaedic management of the Ehlers-Danlos syndromes. Am J Med Genet C Semin Med Genet. 2017;175(1):188–94. https://doi.org/10.1002/ajmg.c.31551.

Falkerslev S, Baago C, Alkjær T, Remvig L, Halkjær-Kristensen J, Larsen PK, et al. Dynamic balance during gait in children and adults with generalized joint hypermobility. Clin Biomech (bristol, Avon). 2013;28:318–24.

Fatoye FA, Palmer S, van der Linden ML, Rowe PJ, Macmillan F. Gait kinematics and passive knee joint range of motion in children with hypermobility syndrome. Gait Posture. 2011;33(3):447–51. https://doi.org/10.1016/j.gaitpost.2010.12.022.

Fatoye F, Palmer S, MacMillan F, Rowe P, Van Der Linden M. Pain intensity and quality of life perception in children with hypermobility syndrome. Rheumatol Int. 2012;32(5):1277–84. https://doi.org/10.1007/s00296-010-1729-2.

Ferrell WR, Tennant N, Sturrock RD. Amelioration of symptoms by enhancement of proprioception in patients with joint hypermobility syndrome. Arthr Rheum. 2004;50:3323–8.

Galli M, Cimolin V, Rigoldi C, Castori M, Celletti C, Albertini G, et al. Gait strategy in patients with Ehlers-Danlos syndrome hypermobility type: a kinematic and kinetic evaluation using 3D gait analysis. Res Dev Disabil. 2011;32(5):1663–8. https://doi.org/10.1016/j.ridd.2011.02.018.

Gazit Y, Jacob G, Grahame R. Ehlers-Danlos syndrome-hypermobility type: a much neglected multisystemic disorder. Rambam Maimonides Med J. 2016;7: e0034.

Gensemer C, Burks R, Kautz S, Judge DP, Lavallee M, Norris RA. Hypermobile Ehlers-Danlos syndromes: complex phenotypes, challenging diagnoses, and poorly understood causes. Dev Dyn. 2021;250:318–44.

Ghibellini G, Brancati F, Castori M. Neurodevelopmental attributes of joint hypermobility syndrome/Ehlers-Danlos syndrome, hypermobility type: update and perspectives. Am J Med Genet C Semin Med Genet. 2015;169C(1):107–16. https://doi.org/10.1002/ajmg.c.31424. Epub 2015 Feb 5.

Grahame R. Joint hypermobility syndrome pain. Curr Pain Headache Rep. 2009;13(6):427–33. https://doi.org/10.1007/s11916-009-0070-5.

Hamonet C, Brissot R, Anne Gompel A, Baeza-Velasco C, Guinchat V, Brock, et al. Ehlers-Danlos Syndrome (EDS)—contribution to clinical diagnosis—a prospective study of 853 patients. EC Neurol 2018;10(6):428–39.

Jansson A, Saartok T, Werner S, Renstrom P. General joint laxity in 1845 Swedish school children of different ages: age- and gender-specific distributions. Acta Paediatr. 2004;93:1202–6.

Kemp S, Roberts I, Gamble C, Wilkinson S, Davidson JE, Baildam EM, et al. A randomized comparative trial of generalized vs targeted physiotherapy in the management of childhood hypermobility. Rheumatology (oxford). 2010;49:315–25.

Kirby A, Davies R. Developmental coordination disorder and joint hypermobility syndrome–overlapping disorders? Implications for research and clinical practice. Child Care Health Dev. 2007;33:513–9.

Kirby A, Davies R, Bryant A. Hypermobility syndrome and developmental coordination disorder: similarities and features. Int J Ther Rehabil. 2005;12:431–7.

Mintz-Itkin R, Lerman-Sagie T, Zuk L, Itkin-Webman T, Davidovitch M. Does physical therapy improve outcome in infants with joint hypermobility and benign hypotonia? J Child Neurol. 2009;24:714–9.

Mu W, Muriello M, Clemens JL, et al. Factors affecting quality of life in children and adolescents with hypermobile Ehlers Danlos syndrome/hypermobility spectrum disorders. Am J Med Genet Part A. 2018;2019:1–9. https://doi.org/10.1002/ajmg.a.61055.

Pacey V, Adams RD, Tofts L, Munns CF, Nicholson LL. Joint hypermobility syndrome subclassification in paediatrics: a factor analytic approach. Arch Dis Child. 2015;100:8–13.

Rombaut L, Malfait F, De Wandele I, Mahieu N, Thijs Y, Segers P, et al. Muscle-tendon tissue properties in the hypermobility type of Ehlers-Danlos syndrome. Arthritis Care Res (hoboken). 2012;64:766–72.

Scheper MC, Juul-Kristensen B, Rombaut L, Rameckers EA, Verbunt J, Engelbert RH. Disability in adolescents and adults diagnosed with hypermobility-related disorders: a meta-analysis. Arch Phys Med Rehabil. 2016;97(12):2174–87. https://doi.org/10.1016/j.apmr.2016.02.015.

Scheper MC, Juul-Kristensen B, Rombaut L, Rameckers EA, Verbunt J, Engelbert RH. Disability in adolescents and adults diagnosed with hypermobility-related disorders: a meta-analysis. Arch Phys Med Rehabil. 2016;97:2174–87.

Schubert-Hjalmarsson E, Ohman A, Kyllerman M, Beckung E. Pain, balance, activity, and participation in children with hypermobility syndrome. Pediatr Phys Ther. 2012;24:339–44.

Shirley ED, Demaio M, Bodurtha J. Ehlers-danlos syndrome in orthopaedics: etiology, diagnosis, and treatment implications. Sports Health. 2012;4:394–403.

Simmonds JV, Keer RJ. Hypermobility and the hypermobility syndrome, part 2: assessment and management of hypermobility syndrome: illustrated via case studies. Man Ther. 2008;13(2):1–11. https://doi.org/10.1016/j.math.2007.11.001.

Smith TO, Jerman E, Easton V, Bacon H, Armon K, Poland F, et al. Do people with benign joint hypermobility syndrome (BJHS) have reduced joint proprioception? A systematic review and meta-analysis. Rheumatol Int. 2013;33:2709–16. https://doi.org/10.1007/s00296-013-2790-4.

Solomon JA, Abrams L, Lichtenstein GR. GI manifestations of Ehlers-Danlos syndrome. Am J Gastroenterol. 1996;91:2282–8.

Weinberg J, Doeriing C, McFarland EG. Joint surgery in Ehlers-Danlos patients: results of a survey. Am J Orthop. 1999;28:406–9.

Younger J, Parkitny L, McLain D. The use of low-dose naltrexone (LDN) as a novel anti-inflammatory treatment for chronic pain. Clin Rheumatol. 2014;33:451–9.

14

History of Joint Hypermobility and Ehlers-Danlos Syndromes in Brazil

Personal Experience of JH and the EDS in Brazil, South America

The history of joint hypermobility (JH) and Ehlers-Danlos Syndromes (EDS) in Brazil has a trajectory of persistence in academic, professional, research and community life, aiming at investigating, taking care of affected individuals and raising general awareness. There have been great advances that motivate us to continue this work, even though persistence is still needed for all aspects, given the complexity of these disorders. In this context, knowledge on the part of professionals is essential, especially of paediatricians and dentists since early interventions in childhood promote functional health and autonomy for care throughout the different periods of life.

The profile of these patients is also another factor that contributes to slow advances. Their clinical manifestations change constantly with many problems since childhood. Moreover, these individuals carry a large volume of complementary exams and are complainers with poor response to medication, as well as being discredited. Thus, there is a demand for longer consultation time, periodic reassessments and continued management.

Despite diverse uninterrupted actions in Brazil, until 2017 health professionals had little interest and/or were unaware of JH and its related conditions. At that time, the few physicians who provided consultations rarely concluded that the condition was an EDS subtype. This reality became even more complex with the New Classification for EDS in 2017 (Malfait et al. 2017). The new diagnostic criteria caused difficulties for clinicians because a new diagnosis was added for the exclusion of the EDS. This was termed "Hypermobility Spectrum Disorders (HSD)" (Castori et al. 2017). This situation concerns among clinicians, since it was expected that the majority of the patients would not meet the criteria for this specific syndrome. Fortunately, this adverse situation did not the case.

For over 30 years, lectures were given to teachers at all school levels, from kindergarten to public and private universities and university centres. These lectures were also given in scientific events and countless interviews by the local, regional and national media, in addition to scientific publications in national and international journals. Moreover, a specific class on this subject was included in the *Stricto Sensu* Postgraduate Course at the Faculty of Medicine of São José do Rio Preto (FAMERP), SP and Brazil. There was also the opportunity to address content on JH and EDS syllabus in the "Collective Health" class for first and second year medical undergraduate students.

The greatest achievement with high visibility was the implementation of the Hypermobility and Ehlers-Danlos

Syndromes Outpatient Clinic (the only one in Brazil), in association with the Specialty Outpatient Clinic of the Hospital de Base in São José do Rio Preto. This implementation was undertaken by the Foundation of the Regional Faculty of Medicine of São José do Rio Preto (FUNFARME), which is an in-service teaching field for undergraduate students in medicine, psychology and nursing, as well as for students of *Lato Sensu* postgraduate courses in different areas of health. This public hospital is a national reference centre in care, teaching and research and is notable for its quality in the fields of health practices.

Activities of assistance, teaching, research and extension to people with JH and related manifestations were strongly influenced by the interest in assisting patients at the Rheumatology Service at FUNFARME/FAMERP. This hospital and outpatient complex provided knowledge and practical experiences that enhanced the curiosity and desire to improve the health of those affected by rheumatic manifestations. These were predominantly chronic musculoskeletal pain and deformities in the locomotor system, with disabilities and/or physical disabilities, which demanded a better understanding of body mechanics and the benefits of ergonomics for these patients.

Proper biomechanics with protection of the locomotor system structures during childhood and adolescence enhance the quality of life for affected adults. This perception was achieved by the coexistence of young, adults and elderly people with severe but preventable sequelae in the locomotor system.

In this context, it is possible to understand how the characteristic of JH leads to derangements in body mechanics, with silent and gradual micro and macro structural lesions, which potentiate the symptoms of pain, fatigue and sleep disorder, among others. Even for asymptomatic JH, it is not possible to accept that this is a benign condition, since the locomotor mechanism demands a regulatory system for the muscle chains to maintain joint and inter-joint congruence. The avoidance of traumatic processes throughout the life cycles is crucial.

Therefore, early physical therapy assistance in the promotion and prevention of JH manifestations, which will surely affect at least physical health since childhood and will improve the quality of life of these patients. These children will be different from the current affected adult population, which has several sequelae arising from insufficient knowledge about "the motion sickness."

My interest in genetic diseases came from high school, which expanded in the undergraduate physiotherapy course. In 1984, I started my activities with the Hospital de Base, linked to the complex of FAMERP and, in 1988 with the Municipal Health and Education Department of São José do Rio Preto, SP. Thus, the actions aimed at people with JH were effectively carried out but are still far from the necessary.

Still in 1984, I started multidisciplinary activities in a private clinic in São José do Rio Preto, also to assist people with JH and Ehlers-Danlos Syndromes, working with a multidisciplinary team for diagnostic support and treatment. This situation facilitated greater involvement of professionals in the specialties, which are also relevant as support for the diagnosis of exclusion and for the definitive diagnosis. Advances in the care of these patients in Brazil were slow but are in progress.

In the general physical therapy outpatient service, which began in 1984, most referrals were made by the Rheumatology Service. These involved different age groups, and the main complaints were of chronic, generalized, disabling musculoskeletal pain with functional impairments in body mechanics. The main initial diagnosis was osteoarthritis/osteoarthrosis, rheumatoid arthritis, and some ankylosing spondylitis. The characteristics were also sometimes present in the family. However, it was known that these were disorders of unknown aetiology, with motor impairment. These, in common, still young, evolved to degenerative processes with little success by treatments with the use of drugs.

In 1985, the Upper Limb Physiotherapy Outpatient Clinic was inaugurated, given the great demand of patients with musculoskeletal problems, such as shoulder joint dislocations and subluxations, osteoarthritis in the hands, and instabilities in the wrists and fingers, with soft tissue disorders, among others. It is now believed that some of these persons had characteristics related to JH.

In 1987, physiotherapy assistance activities began with the Municipality of São José do Rio Preto to implement assistance services for promotion, prevention and physical rehabilitation. On this occasion, health promotion actions were added to 26 preschool units, which resulted in my Master's thesis (Lamari 1994) on the characterization of children with JH. My advisor was Prof. Dr Marileila Varella Garcia, who recently retired from the School of Medicine at the University of Colorado, Denver—USA and who went down in history. The academic career ended with research exclusively on the JH theme, both for the doctoral thesis (Lamari 2000) and for Senior Lecturer (Livre-Docente) (Lamari 2009).

Subsequently, a Medium Complexity Rehabilitation Unit was implemented for multidisciplinary care for people with JH. An Emergency Physiotherapy Unit (only one in Brazil) for assistance to people with musculoskeletal pain was implemented, as well. Once again, individuals with JH obtained an expansion of health care. The position of Rehabilitation Manager by the Municipal Health Department contributed to maintain constant actions also for people with JH.

It is worth mentioning that the great motivation and confidence occurred thanks to one of the books authored by Tese Beighton et al. (1983) on JH, acquired at the beginning of this whole story. Later on, more of his books provided the search for specialized scientific literature, which in turn lead to the participation of the "I Ehlers-Danlos Syndrome Symposium" in Belgium (2012) (Lamari 2012) and others, where it was possible to meet the world scientific community in this research field (Fig. 14.1).

In 2013, Brazil hosted the "I International Congress on Hypermobility, Ehlers-Danlos Syndrome and Pain" (Lamari and Lamari 2013), from August 23 to 25 in the city of São José do Rio Preto (Fig. 14.2), under our coordination, as well as in 2015 (Lamari et al. 2015), 2017 (Lamari and Lamari 2017) 2021 (Lamari et al. 2021) and 2023 (Lamari 2023) (foreseen). As of 2015 (Lamari et al. 2015) (Fig. 14.3) the "International Meeting of

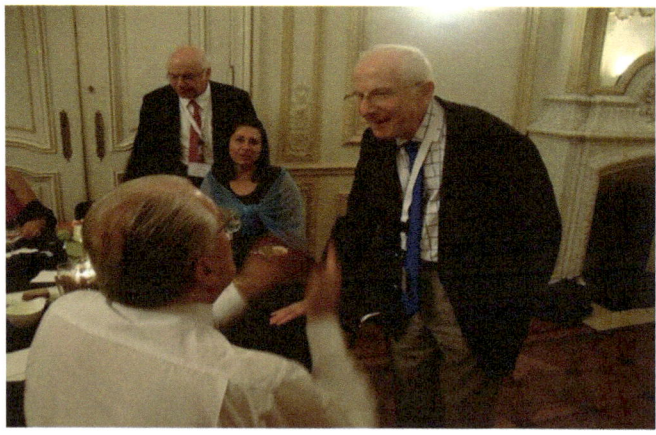

Fig. 14.1 Meeting with Dr Rodney Grahame (England) and Dr Claude Hamonet (France) during the "First International Symposium on the Ehlers-Danlos Syndrome" in Ghent, Belgium-September 8th–11th, 2012

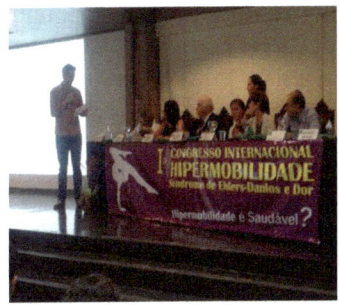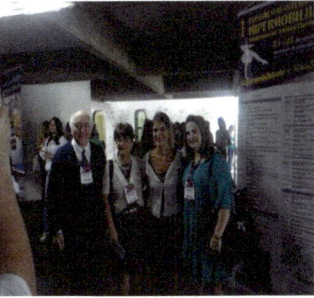

Fig. 14.2 First International Congress on Hypermobility, Ehlers-Danlos Syndrome and Pain in Brazil in 2013 with Dr Mateus Lamari, Dr Jaime Bravo, Dr Marileila Varela Garcia, Dr Fransiska Malfait and, Dr Eny Goloni

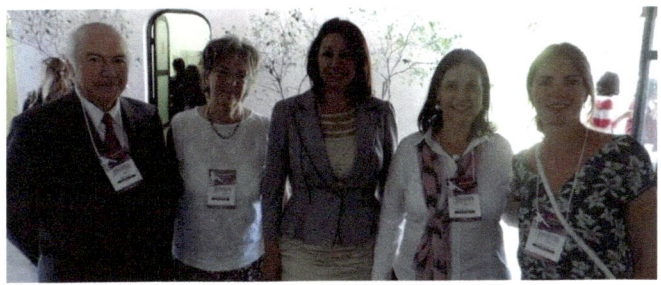

Fig. 14.3 First International Congress on Hypermobility, Ehlers-Danlos Syndrome and Pain in Brazil in 2013 with Dr Jaime Bravo, Dr Margarida Freund, Dr Neuseli Lamari, Désirée Novaes and Dr Fransiska Malfait

Hypermobile Patients" took place in the same period with increasing participation of patients.

In these events in Brazil (Lamari et al. 2015, 2021; Lamari and Lamari 2017), foreign guests of great expression in assistance and research participated, such as Fransiska Malfait (BELGIUM), Margarida Freund (BELGIUM), Jaime Bravo (Chile), Antonio Bulbena (SPAIN), Carolina Baeza-Velasco (FRANCE), Claude

Hamonet (FRANCE), Emily Casanova (USA), Fransiska Malfait (BELGIUM), Jaime Bravo (CHILE), Jenneke Van Den Ende (BELGIUM), Marco Castori (ITALY), Margarida Freund (BELGIUM), Marileila Varella Garcia (USA), Qasim Aziz (ENGLAND), Règine Brissot (FRANCE), Rodney Grahame (ENGLAND), Rozani Lemos (FRANCE) and Lara Bloom (UNITED KINGDOM), as well as the presence of the General Coordinator of Medium and High Complexity of the Ministry of Health. All these events took place always with the support of the FAMERP and FUNFARME.

I was a lecturer in 2016 at the "Annual Meeting—ACR—ARHP" in Washington—USA (Fig. 14.4) (Lamari 2016a), *at the "Ehlers-Danlos Society International Symposium" New York—USA* (Fig. 14.5) (Ehlers-Danlos 2016), *at the*

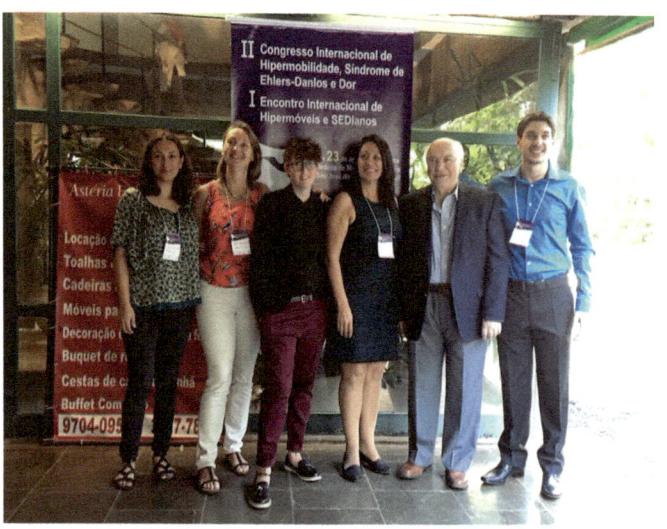

Fig. 14.4 Second International Congress on Hypermobility, Ehlers-Danlos Syndrome and Pain in Brazil (2015) with Dr Carolina Baeza-Velasco, Dr Jenneke Van Den Ende, CEO Lara Bloom, Dr Jaime Bravo and, Dr Mateus Lamari

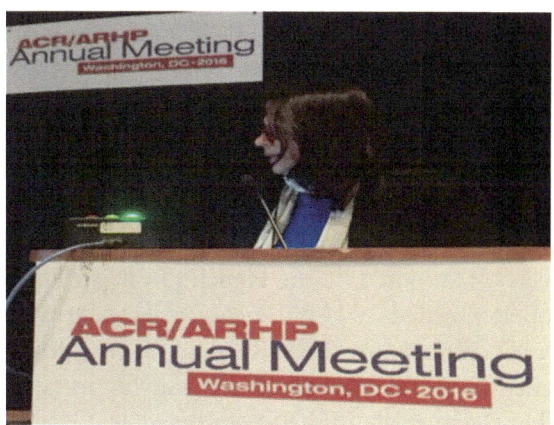

Fig. 14.5   Speaker at ACR/ARHP Annual Meeting—Washington in 2016

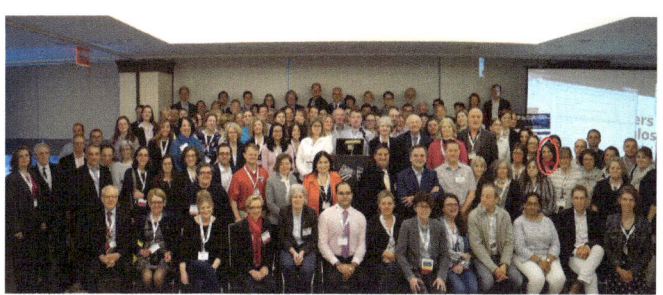

Fig. 14.6   During   the   Ehlers-Danlos   Society   International Symposium in New York (2016) with the aim of reclassifying the diagnostic criteria for all types of Ehlers-Danlos syndrome

"2éme Colloque International Francophone Les Traitements du Syndrome d'Ehlers-Danlos" in Paris (France) (Lamari 2016c) (Fig. 14.6) *and in 2017 at the "Encuentro con Rheumatólogos" (in Santiago—CHILE)* (Encuentro con Rheumatólogos 2017).

In the 2017 (Lamari and Lamari 2017) and 2021 (Lamari et al. 2021) events, special tributes were paid to Prof Dr Peter Beighton, great and eternal mentor, researcher, professor, geneticist. Together with his wife Greta, he established the score to characterize JH in different body regions. The score was published in 1973 (Hamonet 2018) and used hitherto in the vast specialized literature and clinical practice. The appreciation was general among the participants.

The book authored by the French physician Dr Claude Hamonet, entitled "*Ehlers-Danlos: a disease forgotten by medicine*" (Encuentro con Rheumatólogos 2017) was published in 2018, and mentioned and immortalized the record of the history of JH/EDS in Brazil.

In 2018, the biggest and most exciting record in my history took place. That year I personally met Prof Dr Peter Beighton in Cape Town—South Africa. On that occasion I was received in the library of his residence and, from that moment on, our communications became more constant (we were already writing the book). It is worth mentioning that the real library is in him and with him I learned everything. He is an extremely distinguished, admirable person endowed with unique wisdom (Fig. 14.7).

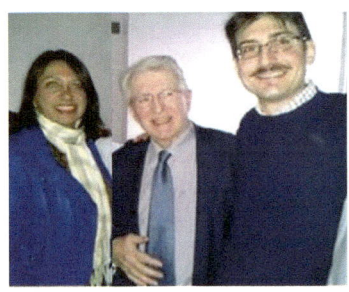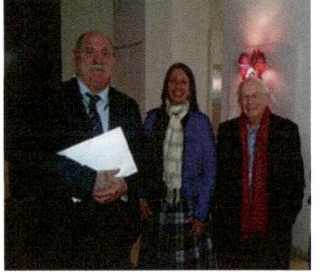

Fig. 14.7 "2éme Colloque International Francophone Les Traitements du Syndrome d'Ehlers-Danlos" in Paris (France—2016) with Dr Claude Hamonet, Dr Marco Castori, Dr Antonio Bulbena and Dr Rodney Grahame

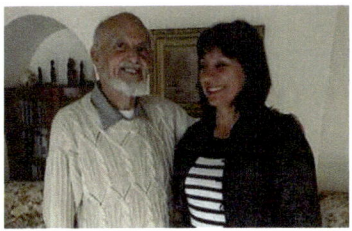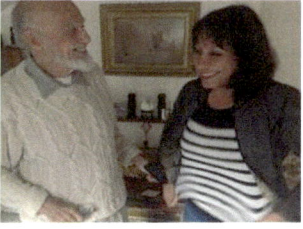

Fig. 14.8 In Cape Town—South Africa (2018) with my dearest Dr Peter Beighton

It is worth mentioning as a continuation of this story, the fact that my son Mateus Lamari has been interested in the subject since his academic life, which took place in 2008 and culminated in his doctoral thesis in 2021 (Lamari 2021). His thesis was published (Lamari et al. 2022). It was part of a large population study in Brazil on "Phenotypic presentation of conditions related to hypermobility spectrum disorders in the life cycles of Brazilians".

In this context, with approximately 38 years of dedication to this population, there were approximately 50,000 consultations for these patients up to 2023. Contributions took place in various ways, directly or indirectly, from lectures in school units for parents and teachers, elementary schools, universities to classes in undergraduate and graduate courses, conferences, seminars, congresses, *lives*, and articles in newspapers, television, etc.: Totalizing approximately 600 actions for the knowledge of EDS. There were several interviews on regional and national television networks, two of them on Rede Globo's "Fantástico" program, in 2015 and 2020.

In November 2021, I received the pleasant news that I was among the three health professionals in the "Rare Woman in Science/Rare Researcher" ((Lamari et al. 2022)

category who represent and do the most for rare diseases in Brazil. It was an initiative of the "Rare Lives Institute".

In 2011, the Brazilian Association of Ehlers-Danlos Syndrome and Hypermobility (SED BRASIL) (Associação Brasileira de Hipermobilidade e Síndrome de Ehlers-Danlos 2011) was created. Previously, there was a community on *Orkut*, which migrated to the *Facebook* group and remains nowadays. In 2012, the SED BRASIL was chosen among eight Brazilian associations to compose the Working Group that elaborated the National Policy for Comprehensive Care for People with Rare Diseases, established by Ordinance 199 of January 30, 2014 (Lamari et al. 2014). In 2012, SED BRAZIL represented the country at the "I International Symposium on Ehlers-Danlos Syndrome" (Lamari and Lamari 2017) in Ghent (Belgium). *I was a member of the Extended Group for the elaboration of the aforementioned ordinance and participated in the scientific event in Ghent. Afterwards, several groups of patients were created by WhatsApp and great advances were achieved due to the efforts of these patients to give visibility showing the volume they represent in Brazil, with* similarities between their clinical and personal histories.

With all these historical records, it is noteworthy that the greatest visibility for physicians occurred as of 2017 with the event of the "III International Congress on Hypermobility, EDS and Pain" and the "II International Meeting of Hypermobile Patients" (Lamari and Lamari 2017). Patients began to appropriate more of the knowledge and developed more autonomy and confidence when reporting their problems during consultations. The scenario now is that of many professionals who are familiar with the disorder. It is a condition that welcomes them, but is below what is necessary for management, definitive diagnosis and specific treatment. Nevertheless, it must be considered that there has been a great advance.

For all the above reasons and from the experiences in different countries, we believe that Brazil is doing its part to extend knowledge regarding disorders associated with JH and EDS. These conditions directly impact the biomechanics and the knowledge of kinesiology in clinical practice of all age groups.

References

Associação Brasileira de Hipermobilidade e Síndrome de Ehlers-Danlos; 2011.

Castori M, Tinkle B, Levy H, Grahame R, Malfait F, Hakim A. A framework for the classification of joint hypermobility and related conditions. Am J Med Genet C Semin Med Genet. 2017;175:148–57.

Encuentro con Rheumatólogos. Departamento de Reumatología, Hospital San Juan de Dios, Santiago, Chile. Hiperlaxitud Articular en el niño y en el adolescente; 18 de abril de 2017.

Hamonet C. Ehlers-Danlos: La maladie oubliée par la medicine. Paris, France; L' Harmattan; 2018, p. 265.

Lamari NM. Mobilidade Articular em pré escolares: uma análise exploratória. Dissertação [Mestrado em Ciências da Saúde]. Faculdade de Medicina de São José do Rio Preto, FAMERP; 1994.

Lamari NM. Fatores determinantes da flexão anterior do tronco em adolescents. São José do Rio Preto. Tese [Doutorado em Ciências da Saúde]. Faculdade de Medicina de São José do Rio Preto, FAMERP; 2000.

Lamari NM. Mobilidade Articular na Criança e no Adolescente: Estudo Exploratório e Inferências Clínicas. São José do Rio Preto. Tese [Livre Docência em Fisioterapia] - Faculdade de Medicina de São José do Rio Preto, FAMERP; 2009.

Lamari NM. First international symposium on the Ehlers-Danlos syndrome. Ghent, Belgium; 2012.

Lamari NM. Annual meeting—ACR—ARHP. Washington, USA. Joint hypermobility in the child and teenager: evaluation and treatment. 15 Nov 2016a.

Lamari NM. Ehlers-Danlos Society International Symposium. New York, USA, 3–6 May 2016b.

Lamari NM. Les orientations thérapeutiques, face au SED, en Europe et en Amérique du sud [Apresentação no 2éme Colloque International Francophone Les Traitements du Syndrome d'Ehlers-Danlos]; Paris, France; 2016c.

Lamari MM. Apresentação fenotípica das condições relacionadas aos transtornos de hipermobilidade em diferentes fases da vida. José do Rio Preto. Tese [Doutorado em Ciências da Saúde]. Faculdade de Medicina de São José do Rio Preto, FAMERP, 04 de novembro, 2021.

Lamari NM. Prêmio mulheres Raras 2022. 27 de Novembro de 2022. Brasil: Instituto Vidas Raras; 2022.

Lamari NM. Quinto Congresso Internacional de Hipermobilidade Sindrome Ehlers-Danlos e Dor e IV Encontro Internacional de Pacientes Hipermóveis - CongresSED. Virtual, 25–27 de agosto 2023 (previsto).

Lamari NM, Lamari MM. Primeiro Congresso Internacional de Hipermobilidade Sindrome Ehlers-Danlos e Dor – CongresSED, São José do Rio Preto, SP, 23–25 de Agosto, 2013.

Lamari NM, Lamari MM. Terceiro Congresso Internacional de Hipermobilidade Sindrome Ehlers-Danlos e Dor e II Encontro Internacional de Pacientes Hipermóveis - CongresSED. São José do Rio Preto, SP, 27 e 28 de outubro; 2017.

Lamari NM, Lamari MM. Segundo Congresso Internacional de Hipermobilidade Sindrome Ehlers-Danlos e Dor e I Encontro Internacional de Pacientes Hipermóveis - CongresSED. São José do Rio Preto, SP, 21–23 de agosto, 2015.

Lamari NM, Lamari MM. Baeza-Velasco. Quarto Congresso Internacional de Hipermobilidade Sindrome Ehlers-Danlos e Dor e III Encontro Internacional de Pacientes Hipermóveis - CongresSED. Virtual, 5–7 de novembro 2021.

Lamari MM, Lamari NM, Araujo-Filho GM, Medeiros MP, Marques VRP, Pavarino EC. Psychosocial and motor characteristics of patients with hypermobility. Frontiers in Psychiatry. 2022. Frontiers in Psychiatry. https://doi.org/10.3389/fpsyt.2021.787822. 2022 Mar;12:787822.

Lamari NM, et al. Ministério da Saúde (Brasil) Portaria nº 199, de 30 de dezembro de 2014. Grupo Técnico Estendido de Trabalho para instituir as Diretrizes para Atenção Integral às Pessoas com Doenças Raras no âmbito do Sistema Único de Saúde (SUS); 2014.

Malfait F, Francomano C, Byers P, Belmont J, Berglund B, Black J, et al. The 2017 international classification of the Ehlers-Danlos syndromes. Am J Med Genet C Semin Med Genet. 2017;175:8–26.

Tese Beighton P, Grahame R, Bird H. Hymobility of joints. Berlin: Springer; 1983. p. 178.

Index